FITNESS HACKS FOR OVER 50

300 Easy Ways to Incorporate Exercise Into Your Life

K. ALEISHA FETTERS, CSCS

With a Foreword by **SilverSneakers**

ADAMS MEDIA
NEW YORK LONDON TORONTO SYDNEY NEW DELHI

Aadamsmedia

Adams Media
An Imprint of Simon & Schuster, Inc.
57 Littlefield Street
Avon, Massachusetts 02322

First Adams Media trade paperback edition April 2020

ADAMS MEDIA and colophon are trademarks of Simon & Schuster.

For information about special discounts for bulk purchases, please contact Simon & Schuster Special Sales at 1-866-506-1949 or business@simonandschuster.com.

The Simon & Schuster Speakers Bureau can bring authors to your live event. For more information or to book an event contact the Simon & Schuster Speakers Bureau at 1-866-248-3049 or visit our website at www.simonspeakers.com.

Interior design by Colleen Cunningham
Interior images by Eric Andrews

Manufactured in the United States of America

10 9 8 7 6 5 4 3 2 1

Library of Congress Cataloging-in-Publication Data
Names: Fetters, K. Aleisha, author.
Title: Fitness hacks for over 50 / K. Aleisha Fetters.
Description: First Adams Media trade paperback edition. | Avon, Massachusetts: Adams Media, 2020.
Series: Hacks.
Includes index.
Identifiers: LCCN 2019054286 | ISBN 9781507212783 (pb) | ISBN 9781507212790 (ebook)
Subjects: LCSH: Exercise for middle-aged persons. | Physical fitness for middle-aged persons.
Classification: LCC GV482.6 .F45 2020 | DDC 613.7/0446--dc23
LC record available at https://lccn.loc.gov/2019054286

ISBN 978-1-5072-1278-3
ISBN 978-1-5072-1279-0 (ebook)

CONTENTS

CHAPTER TWO: FLEXIBILITY AND MOBILITY
65

CHAPTER THREE: MUSCULAR STRENGTH
115

CHAPTER FOUR: AEROBIC CAPACITY AND ENDURANCE

FOREWORD

Looking for a fountain of youth? Look for your sneakers. Then lace them up and get moving. Exercise can turn back the clock, jump-start your energy, and restore your health.

In fact, for adults over sixty-five, physical activity is key to a happier and healthier life, according to a recent study in the journal *BioMed Research International*. Exercise helps protect against cardiovascular disease and diabetes; it also improves mental health and delays the onset of dementia. There's even evidence that exercise helps ward off memory decline and fights depression.

What's more, a Penn State University study found that seniors who lift weights at least twice a week have a 46 percent lower chance of dying from heart disease, cancer, and certain other conditions than those who don't. Exercise won't make you live forever, but it could help you live longer—and better.

That's been the mission of SilverSneakers® since it launched in 1992. Since then, we've helped millions of seniors build and maintain muscle mass, hit a healthy weight, think more clearly, spend less on medical care, maintain independence, make lasting friendships, feel happier, and live longer.

Let's acknowledge two elephants in the gym:

- **Elephant #1: The fifty-plus-year-old body isn't the same as the thirty-minus-year-old body.** True, but that's okay. You don't need to push yourself to exhaustion to stay fit. And the "no pain, no gain" adage? Complete bunk. You just need to move your body a little bit as often as possible. In fact, walking for 30 minutes a day on most days is one of the best things you can do for your health.
- **Elephant #2: While some older adults truly love exercise, many don't.** In fact, 28 percent of adults age fifty and older fall into the couch potato category. Some of us just need a little extra push to make exercise a habit or convince ourselves to stick with it. Maybe you're one of them. That's okay too. As you're about to find out, starting a fitness routine is actually quite simple.

The fact that you've picked up this book means you're ready to make a positive change. Inside, you'll find expert-approved and real-people-tested hacks to build a solid fitness routine that works for you—on your terms, your schedule, your goals.

"If you've become interested in taking care of yourself and trying something new, feed that, and it will flourish," says fitness expert David Jack, whose workouts you'll find at SilverSneakers.com and on our SilverSneakers® *Facebook* and *YouTube* pages.

Interested in fighting fatigue? You'll want to check out Chapter 4 of this book, on feeling more energized. The "Shower at Work" exercise is a SilverSneakers® community member favorite! Want to drop those last stubborn pounds? The fat-burning strategies in Chapter 3 of *Fitness Hacks for over 50* have your name on them. And in the final pages, we'll drill down on the smart ways to stay motivated and keep going.

By the last page, you'll see that healthy living really isn't as complicated or time-consuming as you once believed. It all begins with one small step. And here's the truly good news: You've already taken it. Now turn the page and keep going.

—The Editors of **SilverSneakers**

INTRODUCTION

Are you wanting to lose weight?
Kick up your cardio?
Strengthen up?

No matter how great or motivating our fitness goals, time and (lack of) energy sure have a way of standing in the way of ours!

Fortunately, the most impactful path to where you want to be doesn't have to drain your calendar or batteries—and can be as simple as following the quick and easy hacks in this book. A short walk here, a squat there: These little hacks add up, and lead to a better, more vibrant life.

In this book, we'll move through four areas of fitness that are critical to healthy aging:

1. **Balance and coordination**, in which you'll take a (one-footed) stand; use your opposite hand; or play shopping go-kart.
2. **Flexibility and mobility**, in which you'll relearn to breathe; play air piano; or raise your thumbs to the wall.
3. **Muscular strength**, in which you'll do kitchen-counter push-ups; break up binge-watching; and casually lean on stuff.
4. **Aerobic capacity and endurance**, in which you'll drink more water; take a post-meal walk; or speed mop.

Each chapter of the book covers one of these areas; these chapters (and even each of the hacks within them) build on each other to take you from wherever you are now to exactly where you want to go. You'll learn why each area matters for your health, energy, mobility, function, mood, even sex life—and then, exactly how to grow your fitness in them, without all of the fuss.

After all, most of these hacks don't take much time—often as little as 30 seconds. For lifelong fitness, you just have to integrate movement in your day-to-day, don't-even-have-to-think-about-it routine. Because when you don't need to join a gym, follow an epically long list of to-dos (and to-not-dos!), spend hundreds of dollars, carve out time you don't have, perform exercises you hate, or even leave your house, living an active lifestyle becomes infinitely more doable and enjoyable.

There are also four different kinds of sidebars (Tips!; This Just In!; Did You Know?; and Take It Further!) that will give you more information about the hacks, show you how to do them more effectively, and help you push them to the next level.

But before you start feverishly flipping pages (bonus points if you read this book standing or riding a stationary bike!), it's important to talk to your doctor and find out what forms of exercise are healthy for you. For example, if you have a history of heart disease, you may need to stick to this book's lower-intensity hacks. If you have diabetic neuropathy, avoiding plyometric exercises such as hops and jumps will help your feet stay happy. You may or may not end up performing every hack in this book— and that's okay! The goal is to find a way to stay moving that works for you.

When you discover how to make fitness mesh seamlessly into your regular 24 hours at a pace that fits your age—and your lifestyle—that's when true health happens!

WHAT TO HAVE ON HAND

Another piece of good news is that the majority of the hacks require zero equipment, and for the ones that do, random stuff around your house will usually do the job. I recommend purchasing a good pair of athletic shoes from an athletics store that can help you find the right fit for your foot type.

Some of the hacks in this book require resistance bands (the two types you'll need are shown here), which are a great way to challenge your body with minimal equipment. The bands are color-coded, so you can adjust how much resistance you're using to challenge your body.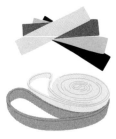

If you're doing a hack for the first time, it's best to use a light band; gradually, as you build strength, move to the heavier bands. You can find them online or at athletic equipment stores.

Ready? Turn the page and become
a healthier, happier you.

CHAPTER 1

BALANCE AND COORDINATION

Balance and coordination are the foundation of fitness, improving your ability to engage in activities and exercises that will make you stronger and faster, decrease your risk of chronic disease, and lengthen your lease on life.

But here's the cool thing about balance and coordination: They are as much mental as they are physical. After all, your nervous system—including your brain, spinal cord, vestibular system (your balance control center, which includes the inner ear), and specialized cells throughout your muscles—is in charge of orchestrating every move your body makes. It's also in charge of your reaction time, plays a huge role in agility, and is constantly working, whether or not you're thinking about it.

Go ahead and touch your finger to your nose. The fact that you pulled it off, and didn't poke yourself in the eye, is due to proprioception—your innate ability to know how your body is moving in space and time. It's just one example of how your brain and body are intricately linked.

However, research shows that, over the decades, that link can get a bit rusty, making it more difficult to coordinate complicated movements and stay stable on our feet. That's one huge reason that every year, falls are a leading cause of injury and disability in older adults worldwide. In the United States alone, more than one in three adults ages sixty-five and older fall every year.

Time to get out the de-ruster!

1

Take an Active Foot

IT'LL COME IN HANDY To improve your feet's proprioceptive abilities and, when performed during the exercises in this book, balance and foot strength.

YOU'LL NEED	TIME INVESTMENT
Bare feet.	30 seconds for practice, and then the duration of every exercise you perform.

You'll practice this stance here with bare feet, but you can and should use it even when wearing shoes.

HOW TO Stand with your feet hip-width apart and grip the floor with your feet. Spread your toes so that, ideally, you can see the floor between each of them (this may take some work if you're used to wearing very confining shoes). Then, balance your weight between your heel and the right and left edges of the balls of your feet, right at the base of your big and little toes. This is called a tripod stance. Keeping your toes in contact with the floor, press those three points of your tripod into the floor and toward each other. You should feel a gentle contraction in the arches of your feet. Maintain this foot positioning when standing or performing any of the exercises in (or out of) this book.

2

Brace Your Core

IT'LL COME IN HANDY To increase stability, improve posture, and protect your spine in everything you do.

YOU'LL NEED	TIME INVESTMENT
A mirror.	5 minutes to learn and a lifetime to practice.

HOW TO Stand tall with your side facing a mirror and your feet a few inches apart. Place one hand on your stomach and the other on the small of your back. You will likely feel the bottom edge of your rib cage pointing outward and a dip in your lower back.

Squeeze your core muscles as if you are about to be punched in the gut. As you do so, feel your back press into your hand, leaving only a small dip in your lower back. You will also feel your ribs tilt to point down toward the floor. You have officially found a braced-core position.

Practice relaxing your core and then returning to this position as well as holding it while taking deep breaths in and out (the breathing part is tricky!). From there, try to hold it both during exercises and routine tasks, until it's your default position.

3

Play Shopping Go-Kart

IT'LL COME IN HANDY When you're at the supermarket, Target, etc., as a way to challenge (and train) your reaction time, coordination, and agility.

YOU'LL NEED	TIME INVESTMENT
A shopping cart.	Until you check off everything on your shopping list.

HOW TO Let's face it—some days, the stores are packed. Maneuvering around people and through the aisles will be a challenge. So you might as well have fun with it!

Turn your shopping trip into your own little game of go-kart. Try to see how quickly and smoothly you can weave through your shopping course. Just keep in mind that this is go-karts, not bumper cars!

4

Take a (One-Footed) Stand

IT'LL COME IN HANDY For improving single-leg stability, which is critical to your ability to walk, run, skip, kick, or do anything on one foot. Practice the skill when you're standing in an incredibly long line with nothing to do, and nowhere to go.

YOU'LL NEED	TIME INVESTMENT
Just yourself and flat shoes. No high heels!	However long this line takes. Finally, an upside to long wait times!

HOW TO Stand with both feet together and transfer your weight onto one foot. Make sure your weight is equally distributed between the ball of your foot and heel. (Yes, this is the tripod stance we just worked on!) Once you've found your balance, lift your opposite foot just off of the floor. Don't worry; it doesn't even have to be high enough to see. As long as you can feel that all of your weight is centered on one foot, you've got it!

5

Play Catch (or Fetch)

IT'LL COME IN HANDY When you're needing some fresh air or trying to entertain the little ones (grandkids, Fido, etc.), this fun-time activity will work your reaction time, ability to judge where objects are traveling, and hand-eye coordination.

YOU'LL NEED	TIME INVESTMENT
A small, soft ball and a partner.	However long both you and your partner are having fun!

HOW TO An overhand throw can help you catch the most air, but if you have a history of shoulder issues, opt for an underhand toss. It puts minimal stress on the rotator cuff while keeping your upper arm in a position that tends to be more comfortable for the shoulder.

6

Do What Simon Says

IT'LL COME IN HANDY As a way to train reaction time and coordination when you and a friend want to work out together, or you're just playing around with your grandkids.

YOU'LL NEED	TIME INVESTMENT
A partner, and preferably some outdoor space.	Shoot for at least 5 minutes, taking turns on who gets to be Simon.

HOW TO Perform the following exercises, or add your own, as a game of Simon Says. In addition to moving only when Simon says to do so, you'll have to quickly react to "left" versus "right" directions. No worries if you mess up; just laugh and then try to trip up (not literally) your partner.

Following are two fun exercises for putting this hack into practice.

▶ Side Squats

Stand with your feet double shoulder-width apart and your hands clasped or arms in front of you for balance. Your partner will then call out, "left," "right," "Simon says, left," or "Simon says, right," as many times as desired. Respond as quickly as possible to their directions, squatting in the direction of the called-out side. Pause, then push through the heel of your bent leg to return to a standing position and wait for your next instruction.

▶ Z Walks

Starting at least twenty feet from your partner, walk or slowly jog toward them. Your partner will then call out, "left," "right," "Simon says, left," or "Simon says, right." Try to respond as quickly as possible to their directions, zigzagging until you reach your partner. Resist the temptation to look at them; keep your eyes focused in the direction you are moving.

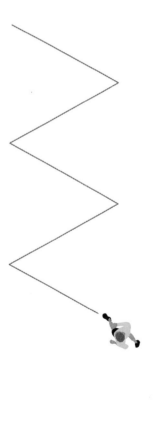

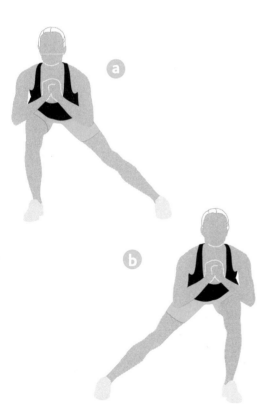

7

Walk the Curb

IT'LL COME IN HANDY To improve your ability to manage your center of gravity and balance as you're walking (the long way!) through a parking lot.

YOU'LL NEED
A stable pair of shoes.

TIME INVESTMENT
The seconds (or minutes) it takes you to walk from your car to the front door.

HOW TO You know how little kids love to walk on curbs like they are balance beams? That's exactly what we're doing here!

Have fun with it, and to help stay stable, focus your eyes on the curb several feet in front of where you're stepping. It can be tempting to stare down directly at your feet, but that can actually throw off your balance. Your body follows where your eyes focus, and you want to move forward, not down!

8

Look over Your Shoulder

IT'LL COME IN HANDY For honing your coordination when looking in a direction other than the one in which you're moving. Try it out when you're walking down the hall or when a cute puppy passes you on the sidewalk.

YOU'LL NEED
A straight walking path.

TIME INVESTMENT
Just seconds.

HOW TO Stand tall with your feet hip-width apart. Look behind you over one shoulder (holding onto something if needed for balance), and then take 4 or 5 steps forward. Repeat looking over your opposite shoulder.

9

Play Mini Golf

IT'LL COME IN HANDY For improving your visual processing abilities while also having fun with friends or family.

YOU'LL NEED Comfortable shoes and access to a miniature golf course.

TIME INVESTMENT Nine to eighteen holes.

HOW TO Keep your eye on the ball. It's a common piece of sports advice, but one that we tend to slip up on as our minds get increasingly cluttered over the decades. Research shows that having a "quiet eye," focusing on the ball at all times, boosts coordination and accuracy even better than does improving putting technique.

10

Close Your Eyes

IT'LL COME IN HANDY When you're exercising in place, brushing your teeth, making the bed, washing the dishes (not knives!), or doing any other safe, routine tasks around the house to improve your proprioceptive skills.

YOU'LL NEED Eyelids!

TIME INVESTMENT As long as you want.

HOW TO Simply shut your eyes during these tasks and try to coordinate your motions sans sight. Use your other senses, like hearing and touch, to help guide you.

Do the One-Legged Pick-Up

IT'LL COME IN HANDY To improve your ability to not just stand on one leg, but actually move around on one leg.

YOU'LL NEED
A messy floor and the ability to confidently stand on one leg.

TIME INVESTMENT
A few seconds.

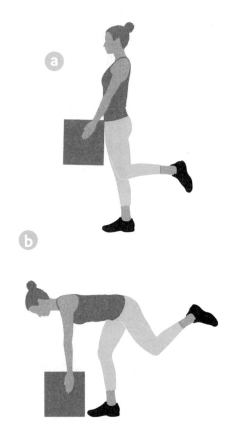

HOW TO Stand tall with your feet together, facing whatever you need to pick up, and brace your core. Lift one foot, then push your hips behind you to lower your torso toward the floor, letting your raised foot float behind you.

Now this is key: Allow only a slight bend in the knee of your planted leg, and don't let your back round as your torso tips toward the floor. Grab the object with both hands, arms fully extended, then push through the heel of your planted foot and squeeze your glutes to return to standing with the object in front of your thighs. Perform an extra rep on the other side.

Did You Know?

This exercise strengthens the entire backside of your body, but also zeroes in on the gluteus medius and minimus in the sides of your hips. These muscles are critical to keeping your hips strong and stable, and linked to a decreased risk of falling.

12

Walk and Talk

IT'LL COME IN HANDY To improve your brain's ability to process and coordinate information, and reduce your risk of falls or injury while walking.

YOU'LL NEED	TIME INVESTMENT
Sturdy walking shoes, a traffic-free walking path, and a buddy either in person or on the phone.	Start with a few minutes and work your way up to fill the length of your walks.

HOW TO Practice walking and talking, sticking to traffic-free paths or at least pausing your conversation when approaching a crosswalk.

This Just In!

Research shows that adults fifty-nine and older have a harder time simultaneously walking and talking compared with younger adults. In one study of street-crossing simulations, older adults who were talking on the phone crossed the street more slowly and were more likely to be "hit" by a virtual car compared with multitasking younger adults.

13

Be the Bird Dog

IT'LL COME IN HANDY If you want to strengthen your core and back or warm up for another exercise.

YOU'LL NEED	TIME INVESTMENT
A soft floor surface.	60 seconds.

HOW TO Get on all fours with your hands below your shoulders and your knees below your hips. Squeeze your core to flatten your back, and look straight down toward the floor.

Raise one arm in front of you and extend the opposite leg behind you until they are in line with the rest of your torso and parallel to the floor. Pause, lower your arm and leg to the floor, and repeat with the opposite arm and leg. Focus on keeping a motionless torso throughout; imagine you have a glass of water resting on your back that you really don't want to spill! Work up to performing 8 to 10 reps.

Do the Grapevine

IT'LL COME IN HANDY For upping your total-body coordination, as well as your ability to look and move in two different directions.

YOU'LL NEED
Just you, and a hallway.

TIME INVESTMENT
Seconds, or, if you really get into it, as long as you want!

HOW TO Stand at one end of the hallway, with your right side facing the direction in which you want to travel. Each step you take will be to the right:

1. Step with the right foot and transfer your weight to that foot.
2. Step your left foot behind the right foot.
3. Step with the right foot.
4. Step with the left foot, touching your toes to the floor next to the right foot.
5. Repeat steps one through four until you reach the end of the hallway.
6. To return to the other end of the hallway, switch sides and perform the same pattern leading with the left leg and moving to the left.

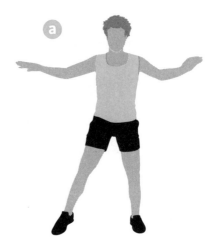

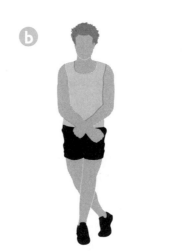

15

Walk the Beach

IT'LL COME IN HANDY When you're lazing on the beach. The uneven, constantly moving sand will challenge your balance, coordination, and ankle stability.

YOU'LL NEED A love for your toes in the sand (or a willingness to have sand in your shoes).

TIME INVESTMENT 15 minutes.

HOW TO Get off of your towel or out of your lounge chair and take a sandy stroll along the beach. The closer you walk toward the water's edge, the more compact—and easy to traverse—the sand will become. For a harder workout, move farther from the water and toward the looser sand.

Take It Further!

There's no end to the number of ways you can progress the Master the Dead Bug exercise as your core grows stronger: ● Straighten your leg as you lower it toward the floor. Bend back as you raise it. ● Keep your legs straight throughout the entire exercise. ● Hold a light object, like a can of veggies, in each hand throughout the exercise.

16

Master the Dead Bug

IT'LL COME IN HANDY If you hate crunches! Also, to activate your core muscles prior to a walk or any active endeavor.

YOU'LL NEED A place to lie on the floor or in the middle of your bed.

TIME INVESTMENT 60 seconds.

HOW TO Lie on your back with your knees bent and directly above your hips, and your arms extended toward the ceiling.

Brace your core to press your lower back into the floor; make sure to maintain this flat-back position throughout the entire exercise. If at any time your lower back leaves the floor, stop and rest before going back at it.

Keeping your knees bent, lower one foot to tap the floor with your heel. As you do so, extend your opposite arm toward the floor over your head. Pause when both your arm and foot are in the lowered position, then squeeze your abs to raise them both back over your torso. Repeat with the other arm and foot. That's 1 rep.

17

Do the Heel-to-Toe Walk

IT'LL COME IN HANDY Any time you're walking around the house and feel like improving your coordination and balance while you're at it.

YOU'LL NEED At least 5 feet of walking space.	TIME INVESTMENT 30 seconds.

HOW TO Stand tall and transfer all of your weight to one foot. Place the heel of the unweighted foot just in front of the toes of your planted foot. Your heel and toes should almost, if not just, touch. Transfer your weight onto your front foot and repeat the heel-to-toe walk for 15 to 20 total steps.

18

Go Barefoot

IT'LL COME IN HANDY If you hate wearing shoes and want your feet to be strong and stable.

YOU'LL NEED To trim your toenails.	TIME INVESTMENT Whatever time you have at home or in your backyard.

HOW TO Kick off your shoes and love life barefoot.

Did You Know?

Each of your feet contains more than one hundred muscles, tendons, and ligaments! These itty-bitty muscles can grow weak with constant footwear—which is why podiatrists call shoes "foot coffins." Research even shows that habitually going barefoot is linked with stronger foot muscles and walking gait.

Reach Around the Clock

IT'LL COME IN HANDY To draw out teeth-brushing while improving your single-leg stability and your feet's proprioception.

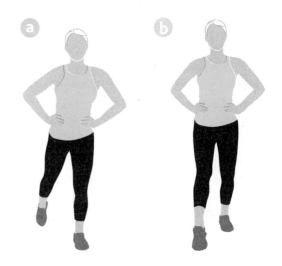

YOU'LL NEED To be able to perform a single-leg stand (aka: stand on one leg).

TIME INVESTMENT 2 minutes.

HOW TO Stand with your feet together and bend your knees and hips to ground yourself into the floor. Shift all of your weight to one foot, and lift the opposite foot just off of the floor.

Imagine that you're standing in the center of a clock, facing 12, and your lifted leg is the hour hand. Slowly move your foot in front of you to 12, then complete a half circle away from your body until you reach 6. Reverse the movement to bring your feet back together. Repeat for up to 10 reps, then try it on the other leg.

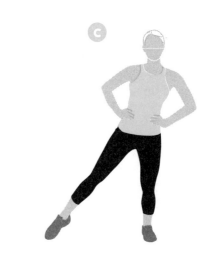

Take It Further!

To make this hack harder, place a mini looped resistance band around your thighs, just above your knees. Try to maintain tension in the band throughout the entire exercise.

20

Switch Shoulders

IT'LL COME IN HANDY If you are carrying a purse, duffle, airplane carry-on, or tote bag to challenge your nondominant side and center of balance.

YOU'LL NEED	TIME INVESTMENT
Your bag.	As long as you spend walking from point A to point B with your bag in tow.

HOW TO Alternate the shoulder on which you hold your bag. Everyone has a go-to shoulder for bag-carrying, and it's surprisingly difficult to keep a bag balanced on your nondominant shoulder!

21

Stomp a Pillow

IT'LL COME IN HANDY When you want to challenge your balance and get in some steps while you're at it.

YOU'LL NEED	TIME INVESTMENT
A pillow.	30 seconds to several minutes.

HOW TO Stand barefoot on top of a pillow (the bigger the pillow is from end to end, the more landing space you'll have). Slowly lift one foot, then the other, marching in place while maintaining your balance on the soft surface. Pump your arms with each step. Progress to raising your knees to waist height.

Tip!

Once you are confident in this exercise and don't need to focus quite as much on each step, you can weave it in during your TV time. March during your favorite show or commercial breaks.

22

Catch Your Keys

IT'LL COME IN HANDY On your way out the door to hone your hand-eye coordination.

YOU'LL NEED Your keys and a free hand.

TIME INVESTMENT 5 seconds.

HOW TO Grasp your keys in one hand and hold them out in front of you. Keeping your eyes fixed on the keys, gently toss them up about 6 inches in the air. Try to catch them with the same hand. Repeat with the opposite hand. It's harder than it sounds!

23

Do the Backward Laundry Walk

IT'LL COME IN HANDY To drill your ability to coordinate complicated tasks on the move.

YOU'LL NEED Shoes that won't slip off and a clear, unobstructed path from the laundry room to the closet.

TIME INVESTMENT 1 minute.

HOW TO Instead of beelining it back and forth with the folded towels or laundry basket, take a few extra seconds and try to make trips walking backward. Keep your eyes focused straight in front of you, and focus on moving slowly and purposefully with each step.

Tip!

If you're feeling unsure of yourself, stick to performing this exercise when you aren't carrying anything—and are on your way to or from the laundry room without a load. That way, your arms will be free to help you maintain your balance.

Walk Like a Monster

IT'LL COME IN HANDY To improve your hip stability.

YOU'LL NEED A mini looped resistance band.	**TIME INVESTMENT** A few minutes.

HOW TO Sit down, and place the band around your thighs, just above your knees. Stand up with your feet shoulder-width apart. In this position, the band should be taut. Take a small step forward with your left foot, then right, keeping your feet hip-width apart throughout. Repeat to walk forward, then reverse your steps to return to where you started. Rest for 30 seconds, and repeat as desired.

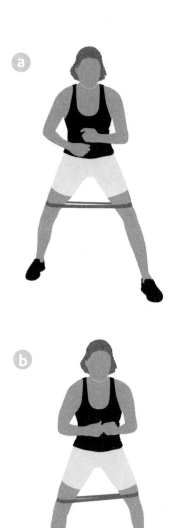

Play Red Light, Green Light

IT'LL COME IN HANDY When you're trying to burn up some of your grandkids' energy and could stand to hone your mental speed.

YOU'LL NEED
At least two players, and an obstacle-free room or yard.

TIME INVESTMENT
At least 10 minutes.

HOW TO Select one person to be the traffic light (you'll take turns); have the traffic light stand at least 20 feet away from the other players, all of whom should stand next to each other in a line, facing the traffic light. When the traffic light says "green light," move toward the light, and when the traffic light says "red light," freeze. Any player caught moving returns to the starting line. Repeat until one player reaches the traffic light. The tagger is the new light, and the game begins again.

Take It Further!

Try these if you're up for an extra challenge: ● Include a "yellow light" command during which everyone must move in slow motion. ● Instead of walking, try hopping, walking backward, or skipping. ● Have the traffic light stand facing away from the other players.

Bounce the Balloon

IT'LL COME IN HANDY When entertaining little kids and as a way to develop your hand-eye coordination and accuracy.

YOU'LL NEED
A balloon and at least one other player.

TIME INVESTMENT
5 to 10 minutes.

If you're feeling creative, use a permanent marker to decorate or keep score on the balloon.

HOW TO Blow up a balloon, tie it off, and stand a few feet from the other player(s). Take turns bouncing it back and forth. When anyone lets the balloon hit the ground, or grabs it with one or both hands, everyone else gets a point. Decide beforehand how many points wins.

Shift Your Focus During Squats

IT'LL COME IN HANDY If you're a multitasker who wants to strengthen your lower body while improving your balance and coordination.

YOU'LL NEED	TIME INVESTMENT
Floor space and the ability to comfortably perform body-weight squats.	5 minutes.

HOW TO Stand tall with your feet between hip- and shoulder-width apart and extend your arms straight out in front of your body. Fix your gaze on your fingertips and brace your core.

Slowly bend your hips and knees to lower into a squat. Only lower as far as feels good to you.

Next, shift your right arm out to the right side of your body. Keep your eyes focused on your right hand, allowing your head and torso to twist as you do so. Try to keep your weight balanced between your left and right foot.

Pause, then shift your arm back in front of you, still following your fingers with your eyes, head, and torso. Repeat on the opposite side.

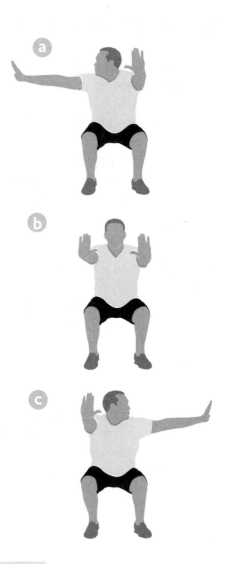

Tip!

If you have trouble keeping your balance, first master the exercise while keeping your eyes fixed on a focal point straight in front of you rather than moving your eyes. Do not turn your head or torso as you lower into each squat.

28

Create an Obstacle Course

IT'LL COME IN HANDY When the grandkids are spending the night. They'll have a ball and you'll definitely challenge your balance and coordination in new, weird ways.

YOU'LL NEED	TIME INVESTMENT
A willingness to tear apart your house in the name of fun.	30 minutes, unless you get really into it and want to play for longer!

HOW TO Use objects around your house to create an obstacle course. Couch cushions, chairs, a rolled-up rug—they all can work. Line them up, and then time how long it takes each racer to complete your DIY course.

29

Get Lopsided

IT'LL COME IN HANDY To ramp up core stability when performing strength exercises with weights or carrying anything in day-to-day life.

YOU'LL NEED	TIME INVESTMENT
A weight to hold or something to carry.	However long you're lifting.

HOW TO Exercise with what's called "offset loading." Instead of holding a weight in both hands, for example, during lower-body exercises such as squats and lunges, try holding a weight on just one side of your body.

Or, when carrying bags to your car, use a different arm or hand for each trip. You'll train your body's small stabilizer muscles, including those in your core, to improve balance. Just make sure to repeat the hack on both sides.

Tip!

Don't let your body lean toward your weighted side. Pretend a string's pulling the top of your head toward the ceiling, as tall as tall can be.

Lunge Two Ways

IT'LL COME IN HANDY To improve your single-leg balance and ankle stability.

YOU'LL NEED
A few square feet of floor space, and either sneakers or bare feet.

TIME INVESTMENT
5 minutes.

HOW TO Stand tall with your feet hip-width apart and clasp your hands in front of your chest. You can also place one hand on a sturdy object next to you for balance. From here, leading with your right leg, lunge backward, then sideways. That's one rep. Repeat with the opposite leg. Work up to performing 5 reps per leg, alternating sides between each rep.

▶ **Lunge Forward**

Take an exaggerated step in front of you with one foot, allowing your back foot's heel to hover above the floor. Once you feel balanced between both feet, slowly bend your hips and knees to lower your torso as far as comfortable toward the floor. Pause, then press through your front foot to step back to a standing position.

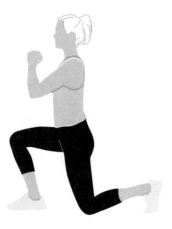

▶ **Lunge Backward**

Take an exaggerated step behind you with one foot, allowing your back foot's heel to hover above the floor. Once you feel balanced between both feet, slowly bend your hips and knees to lower your torso as far as comfortable toward the floor. Pause, then press through your front foot to step back to a standing position.

Tip!

You've probably heard that you need to keep your knees behind your toes during lunges. That's not 100 percent true! Every time you take the stairs or sit down on the toilet, your knees move past your toes. Instead, focus on not allowing your weight to shift forward onto your front foot's toes. Keeping your weight in your heel and mid-foot takes excess stress off of the knee.

31

Skip This Way

IT'LL COME IN HANDY To improve coordination, single-leg balance, and perk up your mood while you're at it.

YOU'LL NEED Just yourself and some room to roam.

TIME INVESTMENT Seconds to minutes.

HOW TO Instead of walking where you need to go, skip!

32

Switch Up Your Sneakers

IT'LL COME IN HANDY For keeping the muscles of your feet balanced and strong, and you stable.

YOU'LL NEED At least two pairs of well-fitting, stable athletic shoes.

TIME INVESTMENT You'll need to spend some time up front shopping, but then you'll be good to go.

HOW TO Even if you have a favorite pair, frequently switch up the shoes you wear. That's especially true for walkers and joggers. Maybe alternate days or dub one pair for weekday excursions and the other for weekends—whatever works for you.

This Just In!

Regularly rotating through multiple pairs of shoes (instead of wearing the same ones all of the time) may reduce your risk of aches and pains—anywhere in your body. For example, in one study of runners, those who rotated among multiple running shoes were 39 percent less likely to get injured compared with those who ran in the same shoes all of the time.

Hitch Your Hip

IT'LL COME IN HANDY For improving your hip stability and reducing the risk of everyday falls as well as exercise-related aches and pains.

YOU'LL NEED
A step or raised surface.

TIME INVESTMENT
60 seconds.

HOW TO Perform the hip hitch, a physical therapy favorite. Stand tall on the edge of a step or other raised surface, and transfer your body weight to one leg. Let the other leg hang off of the edge of the surface, and keep both feet in line with each other.

From here, with the planted leg fully straight, lower your hanging foot a few inches toward the floor by lowering that side's hip. Pause, then raise the hip until the hanging foot is just higher than the planted one. That's one rep. Work up to 10 reps per side.

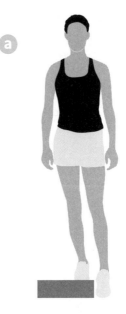

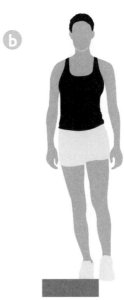

34

Hop on One Foot

IT'LL COME IN HANDY When you want to take your balance and stability to the next level.

YOU'LL NEED	TIME INVESTMENT
The ability to perform single-leg stands, pain-free knees and ankles, and stable shoes.	30 seconds.

You can also go barefoot!

HOW TO Stand with both feet together and transfer your weight onto one foot. Make sure that your weight is equally distributed between the ball of your foot and your heel. Once you've found your balance, lift your opposite foot just off of the floor and hop up and down, trying to minimize how often you have to touch your lifted foot to the floor for balance.

This Just In!

Single-leg hops improve bone strength in a big way. In one study, when postmenopausal women did up to 4 rounds of 20 single-leg hops per day, they increased the bone strength of their tibia (the main bone of the lower leg) by 7 percent in just three months!

35

Pick Up with Your Feet

IT'LL COME IN HANDY If you want the pedidexterity of a chimp.

YOU'LL NEED	TIME INVESTMENT
Patience.	10 to 15 seconds.

HOW TO Instead of bending down every time you need to pick up something small from the floor, try using your toes to pick it up. This will be much easier (but still challenging!) from a seated position, but if you really want to up the ante, you can pick things up with one foot while standing on the other. Talk about balance!

36

Toss Around the Disc

IT'LL COME IN HANDY For improving reaction time and hand-eye coordination.

YOU'LL NEED
A Frisbee, at least one playmate, and an open yard.

TIME INVESTMENT
10-ish minutes.

HOW TO Playing a game of Frisbee with the family is a fun way to improve coordination and agility! Follow these steps for a perfect toss:

1. Grab the Frisbee with your thumb on top, index finger running along the edge, and fingers folded underneath the disc.
2. Stand with your legs staggered, your throwing side's foot forward and pointed at your target, and your opposite foot back and perpendicular to your target.
3. Curl your wrist to bring the disc toward the inside of your forearm and wrap your arm around the front of your torso.
4. Quickly extend your arm in front of you, letting go of the Frisbee with a strong flick of the wrist when your arm is almost straight and the disc is pointed toward your target.

37

Throw Away Your Trash

IT'LL COME IN HANDY When you've got trash or recycling to discard and a yearning to improve your coordination.

YOU'LL NEED
The aforementioned trash/recycling and a corresponding, open-top bin.

TIME INVESTMENT
3 seconds (or longer, if you miss).

HOW TO Standing or sitting a few feet away from a bin, try to under- or overhand toss your trash into it. If you miss, it's on you to get up, bend down, get your trash, and put it where it belongs.

Take a Dance Class

IT'LL COME IN HANDY As a fun way to work your coordination, get your heart rate up, and have fun on date night or girls' night out.

YOU'LL NEED	TIME INVESTMENT
Dancing shoes!	Most classes run for 30 to 90 minutes.

Your usual sneakers will likely work just fine, but Zumba and dance shoes have less traction to help you more easily pivot and slide your feet across the floor more.

HOW TO Log on to Groupon.com or Dabble.co, or check out your local YMCA or YWCA, to see if any available dance classes near you spike your interest.

Do the Side Shuffle

IT'LL COME IN HANDY For improving side-to-side balance and your ability to smoothly change directions.

YOU'LL NEED	TIME INVESTMENT
Yourself and either stable shoes or bare feet.	Up to 60 seconds.

HOW TO Stand with your feet shoulder-width apart and ground yourself by just slightly bending your hips and knees. Hold your arms out in front of you for balance. Shuffle your feet to the right for several steps, then back to the left, and repeat.

40

Use Your Opposite Hand

IT'LL COME IN HANDY To hone your mental sharpness and nervous system's ability to coordinate complicated movements.

YOU'LL NEED	TIME INVESTMENT
A sense of humor.	30 seconds here and there.

HOW TO Use your nondominant hand in everyday situations. This could be when you're brushing your teeth, thumbing through paperwork, or putting away silverware. It will take a lot of concentration at first, but over time, it will become easier and you won't feel so clumsy!

Did You Know?

Every time your brain tells your muscles to take action, it's setting down tire tracks in the snow—allowing for future actions to be easier, faster, and more automatic. The tire tracks for your dominant hand are well laid! For your opposite hand? Not so much. Forcing your brain to lay down new tracks will not only benefit your nondominant side, but also promote your brain's neuroplasticity and ability to grow and improve, no matter your age.

41

Clean Across the Floor

IT'LL COME IN HANDY If you want to train your balance—and if you have a hardwood or tile floor that needs a good spot cleaning.

YOU'LL NEED	TIME INVESTMENT
To be at home with paper towels, rags, or Swiffer pads, and cleaning solution.	5 minutes.

HOW TO Wet your cleaning material of choice, place it on the floor, and step one foot on the material. Use your foot to wipe up small messes, keeping the bulk of your weight in your noncleaning leg for balance.

Take It Further!

Step both feet on paper towels, rags, or Swiffer pads. You'll work your balance at least twice as hard. Just make sure that you keep your feet hip-width apart at all times so that you don't end up sliding into the splits!

Step Wide, Rise, and Hold

IT'LL COME IN HANDY For improving your stability when shifting your weight, changing directions, twisting, and on one leg.

YOU'LL NEED
Sturdy shoes or bare feet, and the ability to comfortably perform single-leg stands and hops.

TIME INVESTMENT
2 minutes.

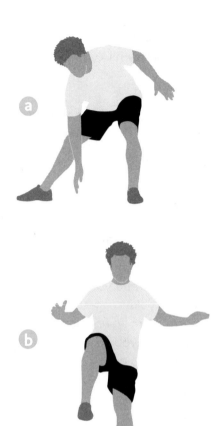

HOW TO Stand tall with your feet hip-width apart and core braced. Step your right leg back and to the right, then bend your hips and left knee to lower down into a shallow lunge, twisting your torso to reach your right hand toward your left foot as you do so.

Drive through your left leg to reverse the movement and come to a single-leg standing position, balancing on a straight left leg with your right knee raised to hip height. Immediately lower into the next rep. Work up to performing 10 reps before repeating on the opposite side.

Get Bendy with Balance Poses

IT'LL COME IN HANDY To enjoy a gentle stretch while you work on your balance.

YOU'LL NEED	TIME INVESTMENT
Bare feet.	10 minutes.

HOW TO Perform yoga's Standing Backbend and Warrior II.

▶ Standing Backbend

Stand tall with your feet hip-width apart, and extend your arms overhead. Place your palms together, and relax your shoulders down and away from your ears. Lift your chest and push your hips forward to gently arch your back, leading behind you with your hands and crown of your head. Move as far into the bend as is comfortable on your lower back.

Hold for up to 15 seconds, then squeeze your glutes to return to standing.

▶ Warrior II

Stand tall with your feet together and arms at your sides. Step your feet apart into a wide lunge, keeping the heels of both feet in line with each other. Rotate your back foot 90 degrees out to the side, pressing through the outside edge of your foot to keep the back leg long and extended. Bend your front knee directly over your ankle to sink your torso toward the floor, and extend your arms out straight to your sides.

Squeeze your glutes to keep both hips, knees, feet, shoulders, and arms in one straight line. Hold this position for up to 30 seconds, then lower your arms, straighten your front knee, and step your feet together. Repeat on the opposite side.

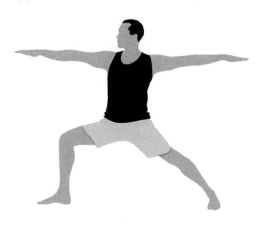

Chop It

IT'LL COME IN HANDY For improving core stability and your ability to stay balanced when you're looking around.

YOU'LL NEED
A small, weighted object such as a book, can of soup, purse, or carton of milk.

TIME INVESTMENT
60 seconds.

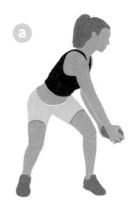

HOW TO Stand with your feet between hip- and shoulder-width apart and hold a small, weighted object with both hands. Lower down into a shallow squat and turn your torso to hold the weight outside of one knee.

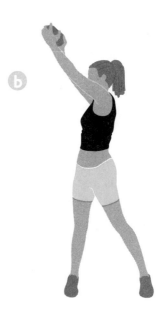

Stand up while raising the weight diagonally up and across your body until it's above your opposite shoulder and your torso is turned in that direction. Pause, then immediately lower into your next rep. Work up to performing 10 reps, then repeat on the opposite side. Keep your eyes fixed on the weight throughout the entire exercise. To do so, your head will have to turn!

Be a Windmill

IT'LL COME IN HANDY To train your core muscles as well as vestibular system. The latter provides the brain with info to keep you balanced and includes your inner ear.

YOU'LL NEED	TIME INVESTMENT
A small, lightly weighted object such as a can of fruit or veggies or a gallon of milk.	60 seconds.

HOW TO Hold a small, lightly weighted object in one hand directly above your shoulder with your elbow locked. Push your hips out to the side of the raised arm and slowly slide your free hand down your other side's leg and toward your foot. Keep your eyes on the weight, with your arm remaining completely vertical and stacked directly over your shoulder, throughout. Pause, then slowly reverse the motion to return to standing, the weight still extended over your shoulder. That's one rep. Work up to performing 10 reps, then repeat on the opposite side.

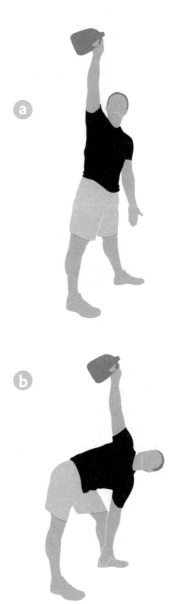

a

b

Lunge and Reach

IT'LL COME IN HANDY When backward lunges are just too easy to balance. Also, this exercise feels amazing and is a great way to stretch your hips after prolonged periods spent sitting. (We aren't to the flexibility and mobility chapter yet, but still.)

YOU'LL NEED A few square feet of floor space.	**TIME INVESTMENT** 30 seconds.

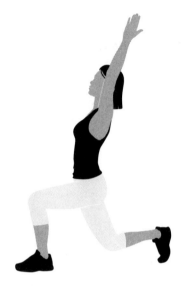

HOW TO Stand tall with your feet hip-width apart, and take an exaggerated step behind you with one foot. Once you feel balanced between both feet, slowly bend at your hips and knees to lower your torso as far as is comfortable toward the floor. As you do so, reach both arms overhead.

Keep your eyes focused straight ahead. Hold for a few seconds, then press through your front foot to step back to standing while lowering your arms to your sides. Repeat on the opposite side.

47

Try Split-Leg Standing Crunches

IT'LL COME IN HANDY For improving single-leg balance and strengthening your core's stabilizer muscles. Also reduces your body's dependence on looking where you're going to maintain balance.

YOU'LL NEED
To have mastered single-leg stands.

TIME INVESTMENT
60 seconds.

HOW TO Get in a split stance with your left leg forward and arms extended overhead. Raise your left knee toward your chest as you pull your arms down and fold your body forward so that your hands and chest approach your knee. Lower your left leg and extend your arms and torso to return to standing, immediately moving into your next rep. Repeat for 30 seconds, then switch sides.

48

Dim the Lights

IT'LL COME IN HANDY At home before bedtime to train your senses and proprioceptive abilities.

YOU'LL NEED
A dimmer switch or the ability to turn off some, but not all, of your home's interior lights.

TIME INVESTMENT
As long as you want.

HOW TO In the evening, dim the lights in your home. This will reduce how much visual input is helping your nervous system balance your body and coordinate your movements. Only lower the lights as far as you feel comfortable and confident; you don't want to bump into furniture in the dark!

Did You Know?

Dimming the lights in the hour before bed can help to improve your ability to stay asleep through the night, which can become increasingly difficult as we age.

Wear a Mini Band in the House

IT'LL COME IN HANDY If you want to give everyone else in your house a laugh while training your hip stability and ability to shift weight without losing balance.

YOU'LL NEED
A mini looped resistance band with a low level of resistance. It should feel easy.

TIME INVESTMENT
However long you're at home and raring to go.

HOW TO Sit down and place the band around your thighs, just above your knees. Stand up and carry on with your around-the-house business (walking, cleaning, getting ready to go out, etc.) with the band in place. It will add resistance to every step you take, challenge your balance, and strengthen your hips. Feel the burn!

Twist on One Foot

IT'LL COME IN HANDY To improve rotational balance and help you change directions, turn around, and twist with ease and zero fear of toppling over.

YOU'LL NEED
As with most things balance, either stable shoes or bare feet.

TIME INVESTMENT
30 seconds.

Try this out only after having nailed single-leg stands.

HOW TO Stand tall on one foot, arms out to the sides for balance, and rotate your torso as far as possible toward your planted leg's side. Immediately reverse the movement to rotate your torso as far as possible toward the raised leg's side. Keep your eyes focused on the same spot or, for an extra challenge, let your eyes move in the direction that your torso travels. Repeat on the other leg.

Practice Your Waltz Steps

IT'LL COME IN HANDY If you're going to a black-tie affair, have two left feet, and need to overhaul your coordination.

YOU'LL NEED	TIME INVESTMENT
Just you. Work up to dancing with a partner.	5 minutes.

HOW TO The basic waltz amounts to tracing a box on the floor with your feet. The leader and follower face each other and mirror each other's moves to stay in step.

▶ **Leader's Steps:**

1. Step forward with your left foot.
2. Step your right foot forward and to the right, in line with your left foot.
3. Bring your left foot next to your right foot.
4. Step your right foot back.
5. Step your left foot back and to the left, in line with your right foot.
6. Bring your right foot next to your left foot.

▶ **Follower's Steps:**

1. Step your right foot back.
2. Step your left foot backward and to the left, in line with your right foot.
3. Bring your right foot next to your left foot.
4. Step your left foot forward.
5. Step your right foot forward and to the right, in line with your left foot.
6. Bring your left foot next to your right foot.

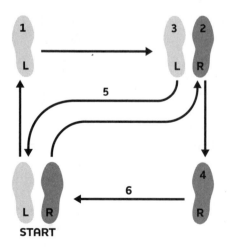

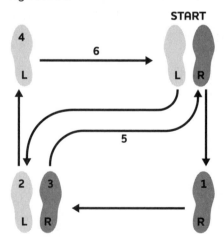

52

Work One Side at a Time

IT'LL COME IN HANDY For added core stability when performing any of the exercise hacks in (or out of) this book.

YOU'LL NEED Whatever you already have on hand for your workout.

TIME INVESTMENT A few minutes.

HOW TO Perform unilateral, or single-side, exercises as opposed to working both sides at the same time. For example, when performing shoulder presses, perform all of your reps on one side, then the other. The same goes for rows, biceps curls, glute bridges, push-ups, whatever!

Did You Know?

Research shows that single-side exercises train the core muscles to a significantly greater degree than two-sided ones do. The result: better stability in everything you do.

53

Play Twister

IT'LL COME IN HANDY To hone balance, coordination, and cognitive processing—all in the name of fun.

YOU'LL NEED A Twister game and a few fellow players.

TIME INVESTMENT As long as you want.

HOW TO Break out the game and get playing! You can play with the official rules or use your own. The important thing is to focus on coordinating hand, foot, and color without falling!

54

Play Freeze

IT'LL COME IN HANDY To train reaction time, balance, and coordination while pranking everyone else in the house.

YOU'LL NEED	TIME INVESTMENT
To be at home with at least one other person.	Consider this game ongoing to make it really interesting!

HOW TO If and when, at any time, anyone in your home yells "Freeze!" everyone else has to stop what they are doing that second, until whoever yelled "freeze" says you can "thaw." Depending on what position you have to freeze in, this could get really complicated!

55

Don't Step on a Crack

IT'LL COME IN HANDY To improve walking balance and coordination, and reduce your risk of falls when dodging obstacles.

YOU'LL NEED	TIME INVESTMENT
Stable shoes, a sidewalk, and somewhere to go.	Play for a few minutes at a time so you can do other things on your walk, like look around, talk, or hop a curb.

HOW TO Remember when, as a kid, you'd try to avoid cracks on the sidewalk so as to not "break your mother's back"? Well, here, stepping on a crack certainly won't do that, but avoiding stepping on cracks can still be a fun challenge. To best maintain balance, keep your eyes focused a few feet ahead of you, rather than pointed straight down toward the sidewalk.

56

Kick the Ball Around

IT'LL COME IN HANDY As a fun way to improve lower-body coordination and control.

YOU'LL NEED	TIME INVESTMENT
A ball of some sort or, if you don't have one, a balloon. Fellow players are optional.	10 minutes or so.

HOW TO Pass the ball back and forth or, if you're playing solo, try bouncing it against a wall, side of the house, or garage door. As you get more practice, you can try to kick harder, faster, and at odd angles to make returns more difficult.

57

Move Your Neck

IT'LL COME IN HANDY Apart from feeling great on your neck, this hack will help you coordinate your head and eye movements to improve balance.

YOU'LL NEED	TIME INVESTMENT
To sit down for this exercise— if you lose your balance easily.	30 seconds or less.

HOW TO Keeping your shoulders square and torso stationary, turn your head to the left, right, up, down, and then rotate in circles, both clockwise and counterclockwise. Keep your eyes focused straight in front of your face— wherever it's pointing—throughout.

Do the Lunge to Single-Leg Stand

IT'LL COME IN HANDY To keep you moving and balancing in multiple planes of motion.

| YOU'LL NEED A few square feet of floor space and the ability to maintain balance during lunges. | TIME INVESTMENT 60 seconds. |

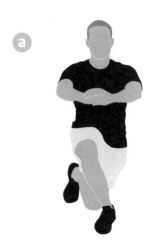

HOW TO Stand with your feet hip-width apart, hands clasped in front of you for balance. Take a giant step back with your left leg and cross it behind your right leg. Bend your knees and hips to lower your torso as far as is comfortable or until your right thigh is nearly parallel to the floor.

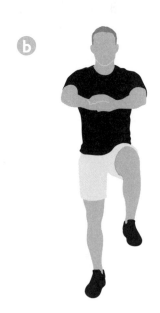

Pause, then drive through your right foot to stand up, simultaneously raising your left knee up toward your waist. Pause, then step back into the next rep, repeating for 30 seconds, then switch sides.

Walk Like a Bear

IT'LL COME IN HANDY To practice coordinating various total-body movements while keeping your core as stable as stable can be.

YOU'LL NEED	TIME INVESTMENT
The ability to get down onto and back up from the floor.	30 seconds or so.

HOW TO Crouch down onto the floor on your hands and feet, your hands shoulder-width apart, feet hip-width apart, and hips up in the air. Brace your core and look at the floor a foot or two in front of you. Step one hand and the opposite foot forward, then repeat on the opposite side to "bear walk" forward as far as you have room. When you're done, slowly return to standing.

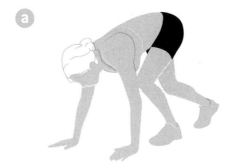

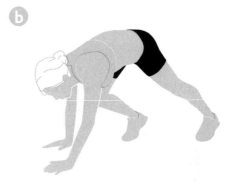

60

Go for a Bike Ride

IT'LL COME IN HANDY For a fun afternoon excursion that will train your coordination, balance (don't fall!), and ability to quickly adjust your path, speed, and more based on your surroundings.

YOU'LL NEED	TIME INVESTMENT
A bike that fits you well and a helmet.	15 minutes or more.

HOW TO Hop on a bike and get pedaling. The more slowly you pedal, the harder you will have to work to stabilize your body and maintain balance. Pick up the pace to make stabilizing easier. Either way, keep your eyes focused ahead of you, where you want to go, and away from mailboxes. Your body will follow your eyes!

61

Focus Far and Near

IT'LL COME IN HANDY For improving visual coordination.

YOU'LL NEED	TIME INVESTMENT
Two objects set in front of you, one a few feet in front of the other.	10 to 20 seconds.

HOW TO Stare at the closest object for a few seconds, then adjust your eyes to focus on the one that's farther away. You should feel as if you're almost looking "through" the first object. After a few more seconds, bring that front object back into focus, and alternate back and forth. It's oddly trippy!

Take It Further!

Do this visual drill while holding a bodyweight squat, standing on one leg, or marching on a pillow.

Step Up

IT'LL COME IN HANDY To take your balance to (literally) the next level.

YOU'LL NEED	TIME INVESTMENT
A step or sturdy surface 6 to 8 inches off of the floor.	60 seconds.

HOW TO Stand tall with your feet together facing a step. Place one foot fully on the step, and press through your heel and midfoot to raise yourself to stand, keeping all of your weight balanced in the planted foot.

Pause, then lower your trailing foot toward the floor. Don't dump any weight into the lowering foot; just let it hover above the floor. Pause, then raise back up. Repeat for 30 seconds, then repeat on the opposite leg.

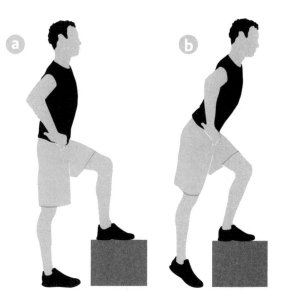

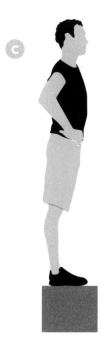

63

Get Mental

IT'LL COME IN HANDY To hone your ability to coordinate mental and physical tasks, and maintain balance even when your mind is on other things.

YOU'LL NEED To pick your favorite balance exercise—a lunge, step-up, etc.

TIME INVESTMENT 30 seconds here and there during exercise.

HOW TO Complete a cognitive drill while performing your balance exercise of choice. Try counting, counting backward, naming objects around the room, watching Netflix, or reading its closed captions. If you manage to do this while also shifting your focus far and near, wow!

64

Wade on the Water

IT'LL COME IN HANDY To practice maintaining your balance and stability under very unstable conditions.

YOU'LL NEED A water float, boogie board, or stand-up paddleboard.

TIME INVESTMENT As long as you're having fun.

HOW TO Water's an awesomely unstable surface. Take advantage of it by trying to keep your balance on top of it—on top of a float. For increased stability, keep your core braced and body low to the water. For an extra balance challenge, move to a seated or kneeling position.

65

Hop Around

IT'LL COME IN HANDY To improve your ability to quickly react to the ground underneath you, change directions, and regain balance upon landing.

YOU'LL NEED	TIME INVESTMENT
Pain-free knees and ankles.	30 seconds or so.

HOW TO Stand tall with your feet together, then hop both feet forward, backward, and side to side. Each time you land, you can pause to find your balance or immediately spring back up to move in the opposite direction.

66

Rock Heel to Toe

IT'LL COME IN HANDY Whenever you're standing around and feeling fidgety, and to improve foot and ankle stability.

YOU'LL NEED	TIME INVESTMENT
Healthy ankles.	2 minutes.

HOW TO Stand tall with your feet hip-width apart, core braced, and rock your body weight toward your heels, then your toes, letting your body lean slightly backward and then forward as you do so. Hold on to a stable surface such as a countertop if needed for balance.

67

Hover over Handrails

IT'LL COME IN HANDY To force your lower body to stabilize yourself when you take the stairs.

YOU'LL NEED To have practiced performing step-ups.

TIME INVESTMENT The time it takes you to go up, or down, the stairs.

HOW TO As you take the stairs, let your hand hover one inch above the stairwell's handrail. This way, you will rely totally on your lower body and core for balance, but will easily be able to grasp the handrail if needed. Note: It may be more difficult for you to maintain balance going down, rather than up, the stairs.

68

Take a Tai Chi Class

IT'LL COME IN HANDY To improve balance, decrease fears of falling, and improve the ability to synchronize movements throughout your entire body. The fun group fitness setting is a nice perk.

YOU'LL NEED To sign up for a class. Check out listings on Yelp.com for tai chi classes near you.

TIME INVESTMENT Most classes range from 30 to 60 minutes.

HOW TO Show up to class in comfortable clothing that allows for freedom of movement, along with stable shoes and a water bottle. Tell your instructor before the start of class if you have any health concerns, but rest assured that tai chi is a great exercise option for people of all fitness levels and abilities.

Take the Less-Beaten Path

IT'LL COME IN HANDY When walking along outdoor paths or trails, and to train proprioceptive abilities to adjust stride, ankle position, knee bend, and more, based on what you feel under your feet.

YOU'LL NEED
Sturdy walking shoes.

TIME INVESTMENT
You can spend a few seconds of your walk, or the entire thing. Whatever feels good.

HOW TO On the edge of most paved outdoor trails or paths, you'll find a few feet of gravel or dirt. Walk there. The ground will be slightly uneven, and even loose, adding a whole new element to your regular walk.

Give a Push

IT'LL COME IN HANDY To improve your ability to control your body against movement.

YOU'LL NEED
A partner.

TIME INVESTMENT
30 seconds.

HOW TO Stand with one foot in front of the other and face your partner, arms extended straight in front of you. In this position, your hands should be touching your partner's outstretched hands. Squeeze your core, glutes, and even arms to make your body as stiff as possible. Your partner will lightly (!!!) push your hands with both hands. Try to resist any backward motion. Take turns, and remember: The goal is not to knock over your partner!

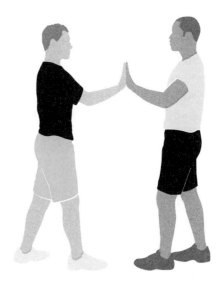

Side Skate

IT'LL COME IN HANDY As a gentle plyometric, change-of-direction exercise.

YOU'LL NEED Yourself, a few feet of floor space, and the ability to perform the crossover lunge to hold and single-leg hop exercises.

TIME INVESTMENT 30 seconds.

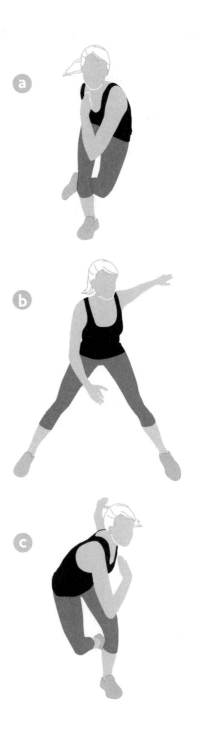

HOW TO Stand tall with your feet shoulder-width apart, core braced, and arms bent at your waist like you're walking or running. Hop your right foot to the right, landing with a bent knee and your left leg hovering above the floor behind you. Let your arms swing. Pause, and without letting your left foot touch the floor, extend your left leg to hop it to the left, landing with a bent knee and your right leg hovering behind you. Hop back and forth for up to 30 seconds.

Resist Rotation

IT'LL COME IN HANDY To strengthen your core's ability to keep you upright when forces, like people bumping into you in a crowded room, jostle you from side to side.

YOU'LL NEED	TIME INVESTMENT
A long resistance band and an anchor point.	2 minutes.

HOW TO Fix one end of a long resistance band to a sturdy object that's around waist height. A pole or piece of heavy furniture will work. You may also be able to close the band in a doorway. Clasp the opposite end of the resistance band with both hands in front of your torso, and stand so that your side faces the anchor point. The band should be taut in this position.

Keeping your torso tall and shoulders down and away from your ears, extend your arms to press the band straight in front of you and pause. Don't let the band pull you to one side. Bend your arms to return the band to your torso, and repeat until you feel like you could perform only a few more reps with proper form. Shake it out and repeat on the opposite side.

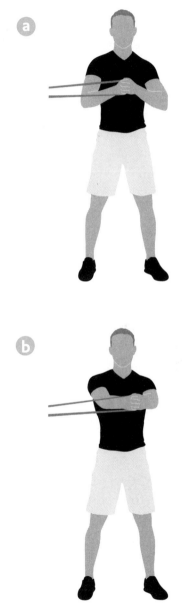

Plank to the Sides

IT'LL COME IN HANDY To improve stability through the deep-lying transverse abdominis muscle, which acts like your spine's internal, stabilizing weight belt. It also trains the internal and external obliques, which form the sides of your core, for added stability.

YOU'LL NEED	TIME INVESTMENT
A soft floor surface.	A couple of minutes.

HOW TO Lie on the floor on your side and place your elbow underneath your shoulder with your forearm perpendicular to your body. Bend your knees and stack them so that your elbow, bottom hip, and knees are in line with each other on the floor. Brace your core and squeeze your glutes to raise your hips until your body forms a straight line from head to knees.

Hold for a few seconds, lower your hips back down to the floor, and repeat up and down for 30 to 45 seconds. Take a breather, and then perform the plank on the opposite side.

Walk on Your Toes...Then Heels

IT'LL COME IN HANDY As a funny way to throw off and train your stability.

YOU'LL NEED	TIME INVESTMENT
Healthy ankles.	2 minutes.

HOW TO Standing tall with your feet hip-width apart, raise your heels until you are balanced on the balls of your feet. Maintain this position—walking around the house, getting ready to go out, doing the dishes—for as long as possible, up to 1 minute.

Lower your heels and immediately raise your toes up as high as you comfortably can, now holding this foot position for up to 1 minute as you move about the house.

Strike a Tree Pose

IT'LL COME IN HANDY If you're working at a countertop and can't seem to stand still.

YOU'LL NEED
A counter, and paperwork or food prep to do at it.

TIME INVESTMENT
However long your balance allows as you're hanging out at the counter.

HOW TO Hold Tree Pose. Stand tall with your feet together, shift your weight into one foot, and place your palms on the counter for balance. Raise the foot of your opposite leg toward your groin, grasp the ankle, and place the sole of your foot against the inner thigh of your standing leg. Press your foot into your thigh and thigh into your foot to maintain balance. If you are unable to balance, lower your foot to your inner calf.

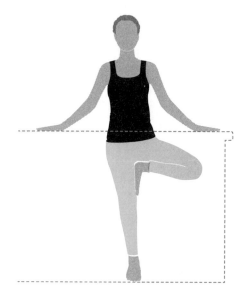

CHAPTER 2

FLEXIBILITY AND MOBILITY

Bend and touch your toes. That's flexibility (or, potentially, inflexibility) at work. Now pick something up from the floor—or better yet, sit on the floor and get back up again. That's mobility.

Did you feel the difference? While flexibility refers to the ability of your muscles to lengthen and stretch, mobility is all about how your joints—composed of not just those same muscles, but also connective tissues, cartilage, and bone—actually move. Flexibility is one of many contributors to mobility, which is critical to being able to move through life like you want, and is linked to longer, healthier lives. It's also mandatory for performing both everyday activities and dedicated exercise with safe, proper form.

Unfortunately, while research shows that mobility can start to decline in your early twenties, most people don't consider it until much later in life when they have a hard time doing regular day-to-day tasks like playing with grandkids or cleaning the house. Recent data from the International Mobility in Aging Study reveals that 15 to 22 percent of men and women suffer with mobility disability by age seventy, with that rate rising to 38 to 62 percent by age eighty.

Where are you along the flexibility and mobility spectrum? Where do you want your body to take you?

1

Relearn to Breathe

IT'LL COME IN HANDY In everything you do, both in and out of this book. Deep diaphragmatic breathing activates the parasympathetic nervous system, enabling your muscles to move more freely.

YOU'LL NEED	TIME INVESTMENT
A comfortable place to lie down.	30 to 60 seconds.

HOW TO Diaphragmatic breathing involves relaxing and contracting the diaphragm, a muscle located horizontally between the thoracic and abdominal cavities. It's pretty much the opposite of the chest breathing that most of us are accustomed to doing.

To get reacquainted with your diaphragm, lie on your back and place one hand on your abdomen and the other on your chest. Taking slow, deep breaths, focus on bringing air into the bottom of your lungs, making your abdomen inflate toward the ceiling with each inhale. Now, keep it going by inflating your chest.

To exhale, contract your core muscles, causing your abdomen to sink back toward the floor.

Once you get practiced breathing this way in a lying position, try it standing, walking, and while you perform any (or all) of the hacks in this book.

Did You Know?

Practicing diaphragmatic breathing helps to brace the core during exercise, improves your breathing efficiency, reduces stress, and lowers heart rate and blood pressure.

2

Slide Against the Wall

IT'LL COME IN HANDY To both test and improve overhead shoulder mobility. It's also a great warm-up move for any activity that involves carrying or lifting.

YOU'LL NEED	TIME INVESTMENT
A wall.	30 to 60 seconds.

HOW TO Stand with your back, hips, and head against a wall, feet placed on the floor hip-width apart and a foot or so away from the wall. Bend your elbows and press them and the backs of your hands against the wall behind you to mimic a goalpost. Slowly straighten your arms to slide them up the wall. Pause, then reverse the movement to return to the goalpost position. That's one rep; aim for 10 to 15. Work to keep your back, hips, head, and arms in contact with the wall at all times, minimizing any arch in your lower back as you do so.

Tip!

When you get started, chances are that if you keep your lower back pressed against the wall, you won't be able to keep your arms against it too. That's okay! Prioritize keeping your lower back pressed into the wall rather than letting it arch to "cheat" your arms to the wall. Over time, you'll get both against the wall at the same time!

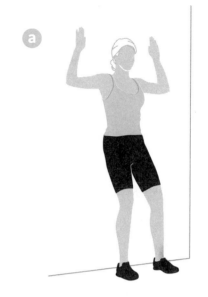

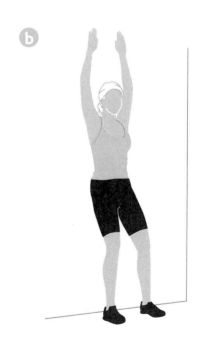

Stretch Your Flexors

IT'LL COME IN HANDY To relieve tightness in your hip flexors (the front of your hips) after long stints sitting.

YOU'LL NEED	TIME INVESTMENT
A soft spot on the floor to kneel.	2 minutes.

HOW TO Get down onto the floor in a half-kneeling position with your right knee on the floor and left knee in front of you. Place your hands on your hips and brace your core.

Lean gently forward and squeeze your glutes to feel a stretch in the front of your right hip. Hold for 30 to 60 seconds, breathing deeply, then switch sides and repeat.

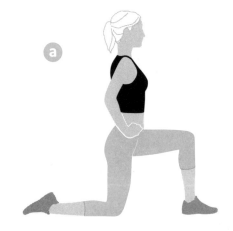

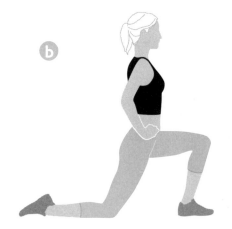

4

Make Your Bed

IT'LL COME IN HANDY To warm up your joints while starting your day off on a productive, tidy note.

YOU'LL NEED
An unmade bed.

TIME INVESTMENT
3 minutes.

HOW TO Hopefully you learned how to make your bed as a kid, but to get the biggest mobility benefits, don't be afraid to do things the hard way. For example, instead of walking around your bed to grab a pillow, try reaching across your bed. Tuck the loose ends of sheets under the mattress. Make it look like a bed you'll love to crawl into later!

5

Strength Train

IT'LL COME IN HANDY For resolving underlying mobility or flexibility issues. After all, a tight muscle is usually a weak one.

YOU'LL NEED
The exercises in Chapter 3 will be incredibly useful here.

TIME INVESTMENT
5 to 10 minutes during the course of your movement routine.

HOW TO Pay attention to what muscles in your body feel tight, and make sure that you are not just stretching them, but also strengthening them.

6

Hang Out in Doorways

IT'LL COME IN HANDY As a way to relieve tension in your chest and improve your posture.

YOU'LL NEED	TIME INVESTMENT
An empty doorway that no one will walk through anytime soon.	30 to 60 seconds.

HOW TO Standing in the center of a doorway, place your forearms on both sides of the doorframe. Take a small step forward with one foot and lean your body forward until you feel a gentle stretch through both sides of your chest. Breathe deeply to relax into the stretch.

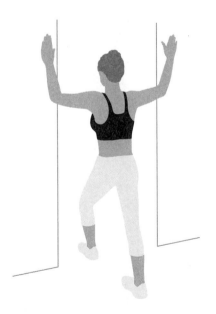

7

Pinch Your Blades

IT'LL COME IN HANDY For improving upper-back posture and shoulder-blade function.

YOU'LL NEED	TIME INVESTMENT
Nothing!	30 seconds.

HOW TO Stand with your feet hip-width apart and arms down at your sides. Extend your elbows down toward the floor and then pinch your shoulder blades as close together as possible. Pause, then release. Repeat, making sure to keep your torso tall throughout.

8

Be a Cat…and Cow

IT'LL COME IN HANDY For promoting healthy levels of flexion and extension through your back and spine, yoga's Cat-Cow is where it's at.

YOU'LL NEED
A soft spot to hang out on the floor. The bed will also work.

TIME INVESTMENT
1 to 2 minutes.

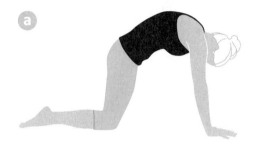

HOW TO Get on your hands and knees with your knees under your hips and your wrists under your shoulders. Let out a full, long exhale, rounding your spine up toward the ceiling and tucking your chin toward your chest. This is the Cat position.

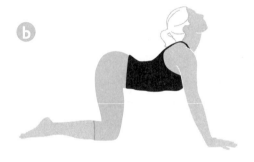

Take a slow, deep inhale, dropping your stomach toward the floor and lifting the top of your head and tailbone toward the ceiling. This is the Cow position. Slowly flow back and forth between the Cat and Cow positions, keeping your movements in sync with your breath.

9

Move Your Ankles

IT'LL COME IN HANDY To improve how well your ankles can move in day-to-day tasks like walking and taking the stairs.

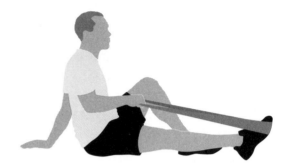

YOU'LL NEED	**TIME INVESTMENT**
Nothing, unless you are ready to build next-level ankle mobility with a resistance band.	5 minutes, max.

HOW TO Sitting down or, if you also want to work your balance, standing on one foot, move your ankle to point your foot, flex it, move it from side to side, and then perform clockwise and counterclockwise circles. You can take turns working each ankle or, if you're sitting, complete the hack on both sides at once.

Take It Further!

Loop one end of a resistance band around your foot and hold the opposite end so that your ankle muscles have to work against the resistance band to bend, extend, and turn. Always hold the band in the opposite direction from which you are moving your foot. This means your hands will move around throughout the hack.

10

Lift Your Knees

IT'LL COME IN HANDY To test the differences between your hip flexors' passive flexibility and their active mobility. In time, regularly performing this hack will close the gap between the two.

YOU'LL NEED	**TIME INVESTMENT**
A wall.	3 minutes.

HOW TO Stand tall with your back against a wall, feet together and just a few inches from the wall. Squeeze your core to press your lower back into the wall. Maintaining this position, grab one knee with both hands and pull it to your chest as far as you comfortably can. You just found your passive flexibility.

Let go of your knee, but attempt to not let it drop from where you had placed it. Try to use only your hip muscles to keep it as high as possible for 10 seconds. This is your muscles' ability to control your range of motion, or active mobility.

Repeat on the opposite side.

11

Reach Behind Your Back

IT'LL COME IN HANDY As a party trick—worthy way to improve how well your shoulder joints and blades move in multiple planes of motion.

YOU'LL NEED	**TIME INVESTMENT**
To have relatively healthy shoulders.	15 to 30 seconds.

Skip this hack if you are currently recovering from shoulder injury or surgery.

HOW TO Extend your right arm up overhead, then bend your elbow to place your right palm on your upper back. Letting your left arm hang straight at your side, bend your elbow to place the back of your left hand against the small of your back.

Gently slide your hands toward each other, with the ultimate goal of clasping fingers.

Repeat on the other side. Keep alternating sides to see how your mobility improves from try to try.

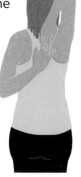

Salute the Sun

IT'LL COME IN HANDY To warm up your muscles and joints first thing in the morning, as well as to ease aches and pains from sleeping on a less-than-perfect mattress.

YOU'LL NEED	TIME INVESTMENT
Bare feet.	5 minutes.

HOW TO After rolling out of bed, start the day with yoga's Sun Salutation sequence.

1. Stand tall with your feet slightly apart and hands in front of your chest in Prayer Pose.

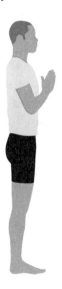

2. Inhale and sweep your arms overhead to Upward Salute. Bring your palms together, drop your head back, and gaze up at your thumbs.

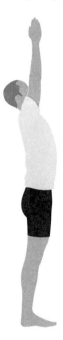

3. Exhale to lower your arms in front of your legs and fold your torso into Forward Bend. Let your head hang.

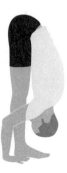

4. Inhale, draw your hands up the front of your legs, and raise your torso until you're in a Half Forward Bend with your elbows straight.

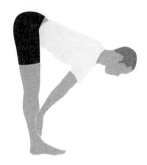

5. Exhale and put your hands in front of you to get into a tall Plank Pose, and bend your elbows to lower your chest toward the floor.

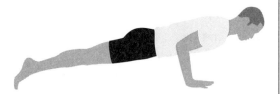

6. Inhale, straightening your arms to raise your chest into Upward-Facing Dog.

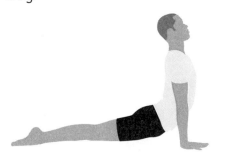

7. Exhale, raising your hips to Downward-Facing Dog, forming an upside-down "V" with your body. Stay here for 5 slow breaths.

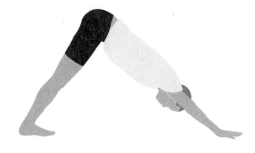

8. Inhale into Half Forward Bend.

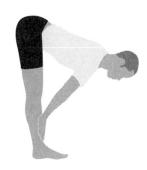

9. Exhale into Forward Bend.

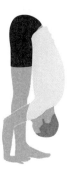

10. Inhale into Upward Salute.

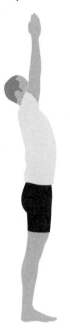

11. Exhale into Prayer Pose.

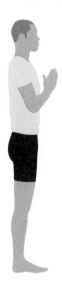

12. Repeat as desired.

Take a Time-Out

IT'LL COME IN HANDY To make sure you break up your computer work with stretching and mobility breaks. Sitting for long periods, especially when hunched over a computer, can contribute to joint stiffness and muscle tightness.

YOU'LL NEED	TIME INVESTMENT
A Mac computer.	Your choice!

HOW TO Download Time Out for your desktop or laptop for free from the App Store, then choose how often you want to take computer breaks, how long they will be, and even what you want to prompt yourself to do during your time-outs. When it's time for your regularly scheduled break, your screen will fade and a message of your choice will pop up and tell you to get moving.

If you're in the work groove, you can always snooze your breaks until you hit a more convenient stopping point.

14

Fidget

IT'LL COME IN HANDY To keep blood moving to your muscles and joints, preventing them from getting tight and locking up.

YOU'LL NEED
Nothing, but an antsy personality helps.

TIME INVESTMENT
Ideally, a few seconds every few minutes spent sitting or lying.

HOW TO Tap your feet, switch up how you cross your legs, shift your weight—however you want to "not sit still."

This Just In!

Fidgeting—also called dynamic sitting—is effective at reducing circulatory dysfunctions that occur with "sitting disease," according to research published by the American Physiological Society.

15

Stretch with Stairs

IT'LL COME IN HANDY As an easy way to loosen up tight calves on the go.

YOU'LL NEED
A set of (non-crowded) stairs with available handrails.

TIME INVESTMENT
A few seconds at a time.

HOW TO As you climb the stairs, pause to stretch your calves. Hold the handrail and let the back half of your foot hang off the edge of the step. Lower your heel a few inches as comfortable. Pause for a few seconds, and then repeat on the opposite side.

Tip!

For safety's sake, never stretch both calves at the same time! You want to have one foot fully on the step (and, again, hold the handrail) at all times.

16

Reserve an Aisle Seat

IT'LL COME IN HANDY On flights, to keep blood from pooling in your legs, and to reduce any aches, pains, or stiffness.

YOU'LL NEED	TIME INVESTMENT
A need to travel.	Seconds to book, and then however long you're in the air.

HOW TO Make it a policy to choose an aisle seat whenever possible. It'll make it infinitely easier to get up, move around, and stretch during long flights. Commit to getting up at least once per hour. Just pay attention to the "fasten seat belt" sign and keep yours fastened even when it's not illuminated.

17

Get a Massage

IT'LL COME IN HANDY To ease tight muscles and improve functional range of motion in cranky joints.

YOU'LL NEED	TIME INVESTMENT
A certified massage therapist and funds to pay the bill.	Sessions are typically 30 to 90 minutes.

Note that some health insurance providers cover massage therapy.

HOW TO Treat yourself to regular massages with a licensed therapist. To check the licensure of your therapist or find one near you, the Federation of State Massage Therapy Boards (www.fsmtb.org/license-lookup) is a great place to start. Going into each session, talk to your massage therapist about health concerns and be open about any massage pressure that is too deep, light, or in any way uncomfortable.

This Just In!

Regular massage therapy improves shoulder mobility in older adults, according to a research review published in the *Journal of Physical Therapy Science*.

Do the I, Y, T

IT'LL COME IN HANDY To improve function in the upper-back musculature, allowing better posture and range of motion in the shoulders.

YOU'LL NEED
A pillow or soft spot to lie down on the floor.

TIME INVESTMENT
3 minutes.

HOW TO Lie on the floor with your neck neutral and your face resting on a pillow or soft spot on the floor, such as a thick rug.

Extend your arms above your head on the floor, positioning them so that your thumbs point up toward the ceiling. Moving only from your shoulders, raise your arms from the floor, then slowly lower them to the floor.

Perform with your arms positioned in an I (arms straight overhead), a Y (arms diagonally overhead), and a T (arms straight out to the sides). Don't raise your chest from the floor or dump any weight into your lower back.

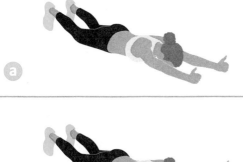

(a)

(b)

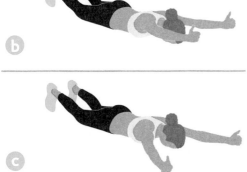

(c)

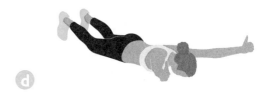

(d)

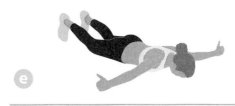

(e)

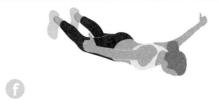

(f)

Raise Your Arms

IT'LL COME IN HANDY To strengthen the muscle at the side of your torso, called the serratus anterior, to improve shoulder mobility and function.

YOU'LL NEED	**TIME INVESTMENT**
A wall.	30 seconds.

HOW TO Take a sturdy stance directly in front of and facing a wall, and place the pinky-side of your forearms against the wall, elbows in line with your shoulders. Your hands should be straight, like blades. Round your shoulders together in front of you to make your upper back flat.

Maintaining this upper-back position, slowly slide your arms up the wall as high as possible and back to the starting position. Repeat as comfortable.

Tip!

If this hack feels "easy" or "relaxed," shake it out and start over, this time really paying attention to keeping your shoulders hunched forward, even as you slide your arms overhead. It looks simple, but if you're doing it right, it's incredibly challenging! You should feel the sides of your torso as well as your core almost "fighting" against your arms.

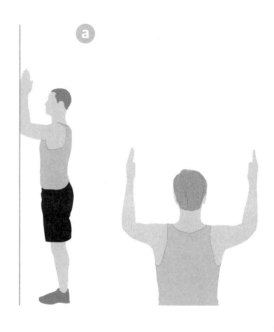

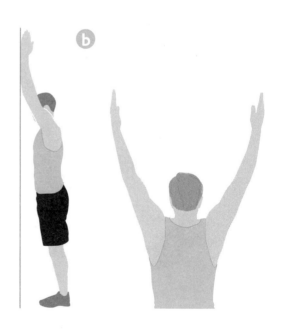

20

Rotate Your Shoulders

IT'LL COME IN HANDY As a way to improve shoulder mobility or warm up your shoulders before exercises and tasks like shoulder presses, shoveling the driveway, or carrying groceries.

YOU'LL NEED	TIME INVESTMENT
A resistance band.	60 seconds.

You could also use a broom or go gearless and play pretend.

HOW TO Take a sturdy stance and grab one end of a resistance band in each hand, your hands roughly double shoulder-width apart. (The wider your grip, the easier this will be.) Let them hang in front of your thighs. Brace your core and, without leaning your shoulders back or arching your lower back, raise the band overhead and then behind you as far as comfortable. Pause, then raise the band back overhead and then in front of your thighs.

Tip!

If you look nothing like the person in the drawing, just laugh it off and keep practicing! The vast majority of older adults—and a lot of younger ones—have trouble accessing this position at first. It's normal, but not exactly healthy.

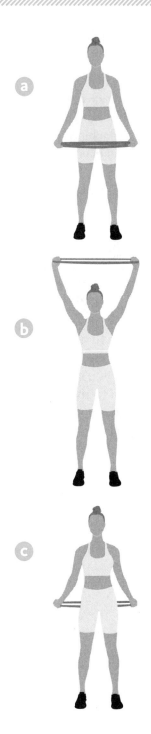

21

Dig Into Laundry

IT'LL COME IN HANDY To integrate total-body mobility work seamlessly into your literal laundry list of to-dos. Bending down, reaching to the depths of the washer and dryer, and finagling rogue socks will work mobility in your knees, hips, spine, shoulders, and even fingers.

YOU'LL NEED	TIME INVESTMENT
Dirty laundry, a washer, and a dryer.	A few minutes to load, then however long the cycles take.

HOW TO When loading and unloading the washer and dryer, pay special attention to how you're moving. Are you able to reach to the bottom or back of the machine without pain? As long as your body says it's okay, try to really get in there.

22

Spread Your Toes

IT'LL COME IN HANDY To keep your toes nice and limber. Remember, your feet are your one contact point with the ground. Mobility there affects how the rest of your body moves!

YOU'LL NEED	TIME INVESTMENT
Bare feet.	15 to 30 seconds.

HOW TO When sitting on the couch or lying in bed, alternate spreading your toes as wide as possible and then scrunching them back up. With each turn, try to get your toes farther apart.

Stretch Before Sleep

IT'LL COME IN HANDY To ease tight muscles and help you sleep better.

YOU'LL NEED	TIME INVESTMENT
Space to move in your bed.	5 minutes.

HOW TO After you crawl into bed, perform these stretches. Repeat each one as many times as feels good and helps you relax into la-la land.

▶ Spinal Twist

Lie on your back in the middle of the bed and extend your arms away from you in a T position. Bend both knees toward the ceiling and then let them fall to one side of your body. Turn your head and upper back to face the side of the bed opposite your legs. Hold for 30 seconds, breathing deeply throughout. Lift your knees back to center and switch sides.

▶ Happy Baby

Lie on your back in the middle of the bed. Bend your hips and knees to grab the outside edges of each foot with one hand. Use your arms to gently pull your knees toward the bed on each side of your chest. Hold for 30 seconds, breathing deeply throughout.

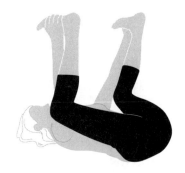

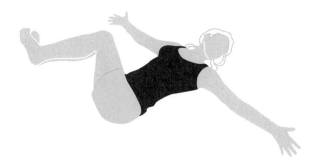

Stabilize Your LPHC

IT'LL COME IN HANDY To ease tight hamstrings. Often, tight hammies are nothing more than a symptom of a weak pelvis. When the pelvis is out of whack, it can tug on the hamstrings, keeping them stretched to their max at all times—and making them feel inflexible.

YOU'LL NEED	TIME INVESTMENT
A sturdy couch and clear (pref-erably soft) spot on the floor in front of it.	3 minutes.

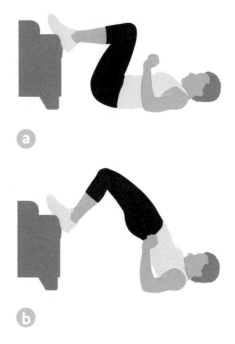

HOW TO Perform the heel-raised hip thrust. Lie on the floor with your knees bent and heels on the edge of the couch, spread hip-width apart. Brace your upper arms against the floor next to you. Keeping a flat back, squeeze your glutes and push through your heels to raise your hips until your torso forms a straight line from your knees to shoulders. Keep your head facing forward with your chin tucked toward your chest. Pause, then lower your hips to the floor.

Continue until you feel like you could perform one more raise, but no more, with proper form.

This Just In!

Research shows that just four weeks regularly training the lumbo-pelvic-hip complex (exactly what you're hitting with this hack!) significantly improves hamstring tightness.

25

Crawl Your Hands

IT'LL COME IN HANDY As a simple way to train both your hand and shoulder mobility.

YOU'LL NEED
Your hands and any nearby surface. (Your legs work just fine!)

TIME INVESTMENT
30 seconds here and there.

HOW TO Place your hand on whatever surface you have nearby and step your four fingers, then your thumbs, forward to walk your hands away from you as far away as is comfortable. Repeat until your hands are as far away from you as comfortable on your shoulder, then step them back to their starting positions.

Try doing this in different directions—forward, to the side, even behind you or up a wall.

26

Get a Better Bra

IT'LL COME IN HANDY To keep your shoulders as healthy and functional as possible. Over time, bra straps can create grooves in the shoulders' muscle fascia, causing pain and reducing mobility.

YOU'LL NEED
The mental fortitude to undertake the challenges of bra shopping.

TIME INVESTMENT
Fingers crossed you find the right bra quickly!

HOW TO Get a professional bra sizing, and once you have your magic number and letter, look for styles with thick and/or padded straps. This will reduce the degree of downward pressure on your shoulders. Regular switching between straight and racerback straps can also dilute any wear and tear to your shoulders.

27

Squat Overhead

IT'LL COME IN HANDY As a total-body exercise to train mobility in your ankles, knees, hips, spine, and shoulders.

YOU'LL NEED
A broom, and some experience with shoulder rotations.

TIME INVESTMENT
3 minutes.

As long as you are holding a broom, and not a barbell, over your head, your shoulder rotations don't have to be anywhere near perfect!

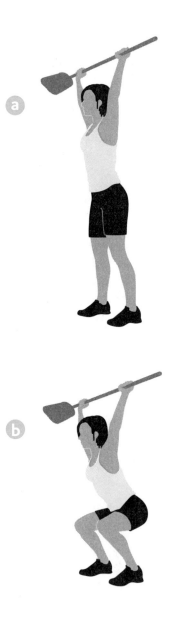

HOW TO Stand with your feet between hip- and shoulder-width apart and hold a broom with your hands more than shoulder-width apart. Brace your core and, without arching your back, raise the broom up until it's directly over your ears.

Bend your hips and knees to squat as far toward the floor as you can comfortably—keeping your heels on the floor, back in neutral, and broom over your ears. (You may only be able to lower a few inches to start.) Pause, then drive through your feet to stand back up.

Repeat, performing each squat slowly and taking breaks to shake it out as needed.

28

Bend and Reach the Sky

IT'LL COME IN HANDY As a feel-good stretch that simultaneously trains hip and spinal mobility.

YOU'LL NEED	TIME INVESTMENT
A few square feet of floor space and either sturdy shoes or bare feet.	2 minutes.

HOW TO Stand with your feet roughly double shoulder-width apart and, keeping a flat back, reach your palms to the floor directly below your shoulders. If you can't quite reach the floor, try scooting your feet out just a bit farther to the sides. With both palms on the floor, take a few deep breaths.

Sweep one hand straight toward the ceiling, following it with your eyes. You should feel a gentle stretch through your middle and upper back. Take a few breaths here, then lower your palm back down and switch sides.

29

Roll Your Wrists

IT'LL COME IN HANDY As a simple way to help maintain tissue health and mobility in the wrists, a common (yet often overlooked) trouble spot.

YOU'LL NEED	TIME INVESTMENT
Just your wrists!	15 seconds.

HOW TO Slowly and with control, rotate your wrists both clockwise and counterclockwise, almost like you are drawing infinity signs in the air. You can do this when you're riding in the car, standing in the checkout line, or have a few unused seconds you want to make a bit more productive.

30

Switch Your Hips

IT'LL COME IN HANDY To improve hip range of motion and warm up the commonly stiff joints before exercise or following a long day of sitting.

YOU'LL NEED	TIME INVESTMENT
Injury-free knees and hips, and a few square feet of comfortable floor space.	2 minutes.

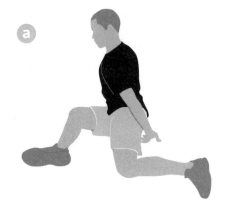

HOW TO Sit on the floor with your knees bent and heels spread and resting on the floor in front of you, and place your hands on the floor next to your hips. Rotate your body to the right, allowing the outside of your right thigh and the inside of your left thigh to fall toward the floor. Follow your knee with your chest.

Pause, then reverse the movement in the opposite direction so that you're rotated toward your left knee.

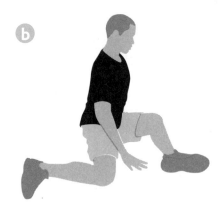

31

Give Your Feet Some Love

IT'LL COME IN HANDY As a way to maintain and improve your flexibility and mobility through your hips and hamstrings while keeping your feet healthy.

YOU'LL NEED Bare feet and some foot-care tools like nail clippers, an emery board, lotion, etc.

TIME INVESTMENT 15 minutes or so.

HOW TO Every week or two, trim your nails, push back your cuticles, lotion up calluses and, if you're into it, paint your nails. Reaching your toes—and maintaining that position for however long it takes to get your feet in working order—will simultaneously test and train your mobility. If needed, take breaks, shake out your legs, stretch your chest, and then go back at it.

Did You Know?

Regularly inspecting your feet is incredibly important if you have diabetes or diabetic neuropathy. Check for any scrapes or sores, clean and dress them appropriately, and if there is any sign of infection, immediately contact your physician.

32

Take a Pilates Class

IT'LL COME IN HANDY As a low-impact way to improve joint strength and mobility.

YOU'LL NEED To sign up, and then show up with water, athletic clothes, and grippy socks.

TIME INVESTMENT Most introductory classes are 60 minutes.

HOW TO If you're completely or relatively new to Pilates, sign up for an introductory mat class to start. Before your session, talk to your instructor about any health or joint concerns.

33

Reach Away

IT'LL COME IN HANDY To work your shoulder mobility while getting everything on your shopping list.

YOU'LL NEED	TIME INVESTMENT
To be out shopping.	It depends on how long your list is… and how crowded the store is.

HOW TO When getting a can of soup or roll of paper towels off of the shelf, don't go for the closest one just because it's the easiest to reach. Instead, try getting that soup on the bottom shelf or those paper towels on the top shelf. (No actual climbing the shelves, though!)

34

Play the Air Piano

IT'LL COME IN HANDY For improving dexterity through the finger muscles and joints.

YOU'LL NEED	TIME INVESTMENT
Idle hands.	30 seconds.

HOW TO Starting with your pinkies, extend and curl your fingers in a sweeping motion, like you're playing a really weird song on an imaginary piano (or your fingers are little spectators doing the wave at a football game).

35

Roll to Crawl

IT'LL COME IN HANDY As a feel-good flow to warm up and move through a full range of motion prior to exercise like walking and jogging, or just throughout the day to stay loose.

YOU'LL NEED	TIME INVESTMENT
A few square feet of floor space and a healthy dose of patience.	A few minutes.

HOW TO Sit on the floor with your knees bent and ankles crossed in front of you, left over right. Roll your hips to the right to place your left foot flat on the floor, and leading with your chest, place both hands on the floor directly below your shoulders. Immediately reverse the move to the opposite side in one fluid motion.

Rock back and forth, each time pressing a little bit more through your planted foot and hands to raise your hips into the air until you're in a crouched lunge position. Notice any tightness in your ankles, knees, hips, or shoulders.

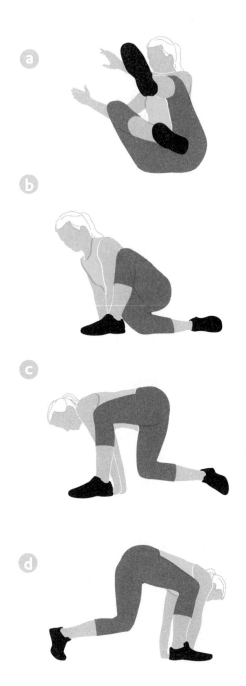

Slide, Twist, and Raise

IT'LL COME IN HANDY To improve movement and function in the shoulders and arms. Here, working each arm separately is a cool way to notice mobility differences between each side of your body.

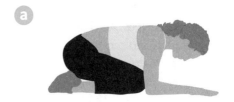

YOU'LL NEED	TIME INVESTMENT
A few square feet of floor space and the ability to get down onto and back up from the floor.	60 seconds or so.

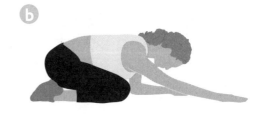

HOW TO Crouch down on the floor on your shins and forearms, heels under your hips and elbows under your shoulders. Slowly slide one palm straight forward in front of you on the floor, turn your palm up to face the ceiling, and then lift your arm up to ear level.

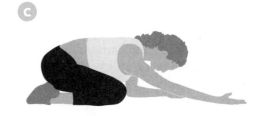

Pause, then reverse the steps to return your arm to the starting position, and repeat with the opposite arm, alternating back and forth as is comfortable.

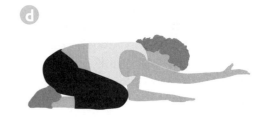

37

Walk with High Knees

IT'LL COME IN HANDY When you're walking down the hall, and to simultaneously strengthen your hip flexors and stretch your glutes.

YOU'LL NEED An empty hallway and the ability to confidently stand on one leg.

TIME INVESTMENT Until you reach the end of the hallway.

HOW TO With each step you take, draw one knee to your chest, pulling with your core and hip flexors. Give your knee a little hug to draw it extra close to your chest. Lower your foot toward the floor in front of you and repeat with the other knee, alternating your way down the hall.

38

Spruce Up the Yard

IT'LL COME IN HANDY To get you moving in all sorts of creative ways you wouldn't otherwise!

YOU'LL NEED Sturdy shoes, and outdoor gardening or landscaping supplies.

TIME INVESTMENT A few minutes to a few hours, avoiding the hottest hours of the day, if possible.

If you have sensitive knees, a pad or towel that you use as a cushion when kneeling would be helpful.

HOW TO Start (or finish) an outdoor project of your choice. Consider tending an herb garden, fixing a fence, planting some flowers, or hanging a bird feeder.

39

Get Up

IT'LL COME IN HANDY For increasing your total-body mobility and function in everything from daily life to sports.

YOU'LL NEED	TIME INVESTMENT
A few square feet of floor space and the ability to safely get onto and up from the floor.	2 minutes, or a few seconds at the beginning and end of any activity that requires being down at floor level.

HOW TO Sit down on the floor and get back up in as many different ways that you can think of. Get creative! Roll onto your stomach, get on all fours, rock on your tailbone, cross your ankles underneath you, do a little jump—the options are endless.

This Just In!

In one study of more than two thousand adults ages fifty-one to eighty, the more easily people were able to sit on the floor and then return to standing, the less likely they were to die during the study's six-year follow-up period—from any cause.

40

Play on the Playground

IT'LL COME IN HANDY When you're at the playground with your grandkids and wish you could still move like the youngins.

YOU'LL NEED	TIME INVESTMENT
Sturdy shoes and clothes that are comfortable to move in and that you don't mind getting dirty.	As long as you and the kids are having fun!

HOW TO Try to "keep up" with the kids (knowing your limits, of course) instead of just watching them do their thing from a bench. Show them some of your favorite playground activities from your childhood.

41

Roll Out

IT'LL COME IN HANDY When you need to ease tight or tender muscles, but don't have a massage appointment.

YOU'LL NEED	TIME INVESTMENT
A foam roller or access to someone else's.	15 to 20 minutes.

HOW TO Try self-myofascial release with a foam roller. Many gyms have an assortment of rollers that you can use to figure out what density feels best to you. Perform 3 to 5 minutes of each exercise. Breathe deeply, moving slowly and pausing for a few breaths when you notice a tender spot or "knot."

▶ **Quadriceps Roll**

Lie facedown on top of a foam roller, with it running perpendicularly across your thighs. Place your forearms on the floor to support your torso and let your feet hover above the floor. Slowly roll your quads on top of the roller, from just above your knees to just below your hips.

▶ **Gluteal Roll**

Sit down on top of a foam roller, with it running perpendicularly across your hips. Place your hands behind you on the floor to support your torso, and cross one ankle over the opposite leg's knee. Slowly roll your glutes back and forth on top of the roller, leaning from side to side as you do so to get into the sides of your glutes. Switch legs halfway through.

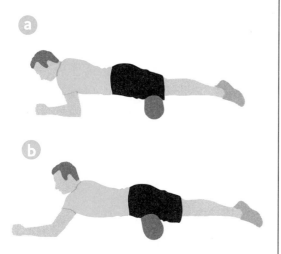

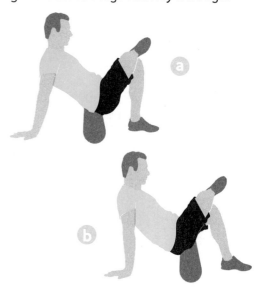

42

Dynamically Stretch

IT'LL COME IN HANDY To prepare your muscles and joints for movement, whether you are about to strength train, run, bike, swim, hike—anything.

YOU'LL NEED
A few square feet of floor and air space.

TIME INVESTMENT
5 minutes.

HOW TO Prior to exercise, gently rehearse some of the movements you have coming with what's called "dynamic stretching." For example, if you're going to go for a walk or jog, practice some bodyweight squats, lunges, or leg swings (standing holding a wall and swinging your leg forward and backward and then side to side). If you're about to work on your freestyle swim stroke, do some forward arm circles. If you're about to try some push-ups, how about practicing them against the wall first?

Doing so will take your body through the motions in a way that stretches and loosens up muscles, but not so much that, like a stretched-out rubber band, they lose oomph.

43

Static Stretch

IT'LL COME IN HANDY Following exercise or throughout the day to relax tight muscles.

YOU'LL NEED
Just yourself and a soft spot on the floor to sit, lie, and move around.

TIME INVESTMENT
5 minutes here and there.

HOW TO Once you wrap up your workout (or break free from your desk chair) perform some classic bend-and-hold stretching. Called "static stretching," it's best saved for after, rather than before, workouts, since it can loosen up your muscles and connective tissues like that stretched-out rubber band, reducing how much strength they can exert, which you need during your workout. Fortunately, afterward, it's cool for your muscles to veg out.

44

Throw Up an Elbow

IT'LL COME IN HANDY For improving mobility through the thoracic spine, which runs from the middle back to the top of the shoulders. It is critical to healthy back alignment, shoulder mobility, and the ability to safely perform overhead tasks.

YOU'LL NEED A comfortable space to get on all fours.

TIME INVESTMENT 2 minutes.

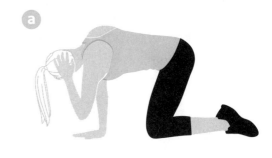

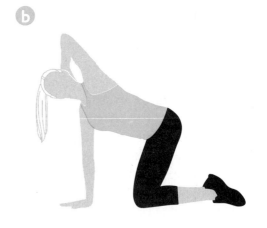

HOW TO Get on your hands and knees. Brace your core, and place one hand on the back of your head. Rotate your shoulder as far as possible down toward the hand that's on the floor. Pause, then raise the shoulder as far as possible to point your elbow at the ceiling, following it with your eyes. You should feel a stretch in the middle and upper back.

45

Use a Full Range

IT'LL COME IN HANDY During virtually any hack you'll find in this book to improve your muscles' and joints' available range of motion. Use it or lose it!

YOU'LL NEED	TIME INVESTMENT
Whatever you're already working with.	However long you already plan to move.

HOW TO Stop bunching up your body and cutting your motions short! Instead, when you perform a squat, lower all the way down as far as is comfortable, not just as far as is easy. The same goes for rows, biceps curls, push-ups, as well as day-to-day tasks like picking up laundry from the floor, wiping down the bathroom mirror, and grabbing your glass of water off of the coffee table in front of you. Use your body's full range of motion, and you'll find that range expanding.

This Just In!

In one University of North Dakota study, when people spent five weeks performing strength exercises, all through their full range of motion, they improved their hamstring, hip, and shoulder flexibility just as well as those who spent five weeks stretching.

46

Dress with Purpose

IT'LL COME IN HANDY When walking outside naked isn't an option, and you need to work on shoulder, hip, knee, and finger mobility, anyway.

YOU'LL NEED	TIME INVESTMENT
A closet full of options.	5 minutes, or longer if you're indecisive.

HOW TO Turn the simple act of getting dressed in the morning into an exercise in mobility. Getting your arms into your sleeves, stepping into each pant leg, getting on your socks, and even fastening zippers and buttons moves your body's joints in important ways. Focus on moving intentionally and with control. No haphazard flailing when you get caught in your sweater!

47

Test and Retest

IT'LL COME IN HANDY To evaluate how your flexibility and mobility improve with regular training.

YOU'LL NEED Whatever hacks you're already using, like shoulder rotations, wall slides, and spinal twists.

TIME INVESTMENT A few minutes.

A pen and notebook would also be useful.

HOW TO Each time you perform flexibility and mobility exercises, your range of motion and abilities increase. Every month, compare how you're moving with how you used to move. Are you able to move your shoulders more comfortably or farther? Is it easier to place your palms on the floor during the "bend and reach the sky" exercise? Celebrate these milestones!

Tip!

When testing and retesting, don't forget to compare how you're moving through one side of the body versus the other. While it's completely natural for one side to be more limber than the other, the goal, in time, is to help both sides move equally well and comfortably.

48

Check Your Blind Spot

IT'LL COME IN HANDY To train your spinal mobility and drive just a little bit more safely.

YOU'LL NEED To be sitting behind the wheel.

TIME INVESTMENT A few seconds.

HOW TO When you throw your car into reverse, check your blind spot—and not just in the mirror. Look over your shoulder like they taught you back in driver's ed (keeping the wheel pointed in the right direction, of course).

49

Scrub Your Shoulders

IT'LL COME IN HANDY To improve shoulder mobility and finally give that spot in the middle of your back a good washing.

YOU'LL NEED	TIME INVESTMENT
Soap and a running shower.	A few minutes.

HOW TO When you're lathering up, make sure to get the center of your back. With a bar of soap or loofa in one hand, reach it overhead, then extend it down the center of your upper back and perform a few circles. Next, drop your arm down to your side and extend it up the center of your back up toward your shoulder blades. Perform a few more circles. Repeat with the other arm. Finally, it's squeaky clean!

50

Double Your Back Work

IT'LL COME IN HANDY To improve your posture and maintain mobility through your upper back.

YOU'LL NEED	TIME INVESTMENT
To love exercises like rows and I, Y, T raises.	Twice as much time as you spend on chest exercises like incline push-ups.

HOW TO Spend extra time showing your back some love. Performing roughly twice as much pulling, or back-strengthening, work compared to pushing, or chest-strengthening, work (both of which we will cover in the next chapter) is a great way to improve posture, maintain spinal mobility, and even reduce the risk of vertebral compression fractures.

51

Play in the Snow

IT'LL COME IN HANDY For building total-body mobility and fun memories with the family.

YOU'LL NEED	TIME INVESTMENT
Snow, and appropriate snow wear.	15 to 30 minutes. If you plan on staying out longer, and the temperature is below freezing, you may need periodic indoor warm-up breaks.

HOW TO Build a snowman, igloo, or get down in the snow and make snow angels. Each will train your body's ability to move in big (often exaggerated, thanks to the snow's resistance) ways.

52

Tap Your Toes

IT'LL COME IN HANDY To strengthen your shins' tibialis anterior muscles, balancing out the calves for better ankle function.

YOU'LL NEED	TIME INVESTMENT
A good place to sit.	3 minutes.

HOW TO Sit down in a chair or on the couch with your feet flat on the floor, spread hip-width apart. Raise both feet's toes as high as possible, then lower them to the floor and repeat. Move slowly, focusing on squeezing your shins to raise your toes, and stopping once you feel a gentle burn in both shins.

53

Raise Your Heels

IT'LL COME IN HANDY To improve healthy range of motion in the ankles as well as the metatarsophalangeal joints, which connect your toes to the base of your feet (think: the balls of your feet).

YOU'LL NEED	TIME INVESTMENT
An elevated surface like a low step or even a text-book, along with a towel and something sturdy (like a chair or hand-rail) to hold for balance.	5 minutes.

HOW TO Holding onto a sturdy object for balance, place your forefeet on the edge of a low step or box, and place a folded or rolled-up towel under the balls of one foot so that your toes are elevated toward the ceiling. Shift your weight onto the propped-up foot and raise the opposite foot just off of the floor. Maintain this one-legged position throughout.

Slowly lower your heel toward the floor as far as possible until you feel a stretch in your calf. Pause, then press through the ball of your foot and squeeze your calf to raise your heel as high as possible toward the ceiling.

Perform until you feel a burn in your calf, then repeat on the opposite leg. Calves are infamous for next-day soreness, so don't push it too hard.

Did You Know?

Poor mobility in the ankles and metatarsophalangeal joints are leading contributors to plantar fasciitis. So, start moving both joints to combat the uncomfortably common heel condition.

54

Hold the End

IT'LL COME IN HANDY To improve function at your end ranges of motion, where your nervous system is most likely to hit the brakes on your flexibility and mobility.

YOU'LL NEED	TIME INVESTMENT
Whatever you already need for your strength workout of choice.	A few seconds in the middle of each exercise repetition.

HOW TO Strength exercises improve mobility. Performing strength exercises through a full range of motion adds to your mobility gains. Now that you have those down, take it even further by adding a controlled few-second pause between the two phases of each rep.

For example, when performing a lunge, lower to your end range of motion, and then hold it. Try counting to 2 or even 3, then rise back up to standing. When performing resistance-band rows, pull the ends of the bands to your ribs, pause for a few seconds, and then return to start.

55

Raid the Closet

IT'LL COME IN HANDY To get you moving up, down, and reaching all around while also making your overflowing closet way more manageable.

YOU'LL NEED	TIME INVESTMENT
One messy closet, and donation, recycling, and trash bags.	It depends on how long you've been needing to do this.

HOW TO Starting in one corner, sort your way across the closet, folding and bagging for donation anything that you realistically don't need or want, and discarding recyclables and dust bunnies as you find them. Leave no region of your closet untouched.

56

Distract Your Ankle

IT'LL COME IN HANDY To manually move the ankle's talus bone so that the ankle has more room to move.

YOU'LL NEED A resistance band and a low, sturdy object to affix it to. Plus, a soft spot to rest your knee on the floor would be nice.

TIME INVESTMENT 3 to 4 minutes.

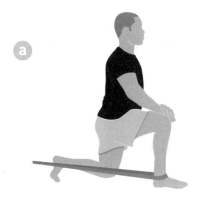

HOW TO Attach a resistance band to a low, sturdy object, just a few inches off the ground. Lower into a half-kneeling position with your front ankle directly under your knee and loop the opposite end of the band around the front of your ankle, right where your foot slopes up to connect to your shin, so that the band is taut.

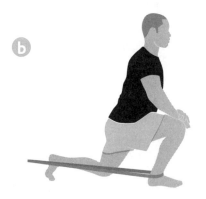

Shift your weight forward so that your knee extends forward past your toes as far as possible while keeping your heel on the floor. Hold for 5 to 10 seconds, and then shift your weight back and repeat for a total of 5 rounds. Then switch ankles.

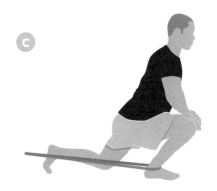

57

Sit in the Sauna

IT'LL COME IN HANDY For a relaxing way to increase blood flow to the muscles for greater flexibility.

YOU'LL NEED	TIME INVESTMENT
Access to a sauna and a bathing suit and towel.	Start with 5 minutes.

Many gyms, spas, hotels, and condominium and apartment complexes have saunas.

HOW TO Change into a bathing suit, take off jewelry and metal paraphernalia (they'll get hot!), and sit down on your towel in the sauna. The higher you sit in the sauna, the hotter the air will be. Temperatures are cooler near the floor. Drink extra water afterward.

Tip!

While research suggests that saunas may improve blood pressure, dementia risk, immune health, and longevity, always talk to your doctor about your health and any safety guidelines you should keep in mind before starting a sauna routine. Saunas are incredibly hot, and you don't want to risk heat stroke or any other issues. Start with super-short 5-minute sessions, and never draw out sessions for more than 30 minutes.

58

Go Camping

IT'LL COME IN HANDY For moving in ways you never would in the great indoors.

YOU'LL NEED	TIME INVESTMENT
Fellow campers and camping supplies based on how much you want to rough it.	Give it at least one overnight.

HOW TO Reserve a campsite and head outdoors with the family. Pitch in with tasks like setting up the tent, collecting kindling for the fire, and preparing meals.

59

Raise Your Thumbs to the Wall

IT'LL COME IN HANDY To see just how good your overhead shoulder mobility is, and then improve it.

YOU'LL NEED	**TIME INVESTMENT**
A wall.	2 minutes.

HOW TO Stand with your back, hips, and head against a wall, feet placed on the floor hip-width apart and a foot or so away from the wall. Straighten your arms so that they hang at your sides and your thumbs face forward. Brace your core to press your lower back into the wall.

Maintaining this braced core position and keeping your arms straight, raise your arms up overhead and try to reach your thumbs to the wall. Hold for 10 breaths and then repeat a few times, noticing if you can get any closer on your later attempts.

Take It Further!

After performing a few arm raises, ask a partner to gently press your thumbs to meet the wall, again, with you keeping your lower back pressed into the wall. How far you are able to raise your arms on your own represents your active mobility. How far your partner can press your arms represents your passive flexibility.

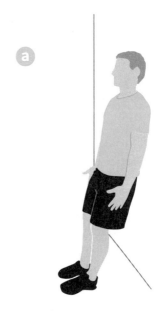

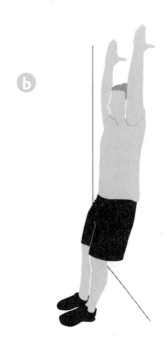

60

Take a Yoga Class

IT'LL COME IN HANDY For a feel-good way to improve flexibility.

YOU'LL NEED	TIME INVESTMENT
To sign up for something new.	Most beginner classes start at 1 hour in length.

HOW TO Sign up for a "beginner" or "restorative" class and show up a few minutes early with comfortable athletic clothes, grippy socks (you can also go barefoot), and a water bottle. Yoga has a lot of inversion, or head-down, poses, so you might consider a shirt that you can tuck into your pants or that won't fall around your head while you're in Downward-Facing Dog.

Talk to the instructor before class about any health concerns or mobility restrictions, and focus on making the session your individual practice. No two people move the same way, and even though your instructor will give you cues and help you throughout, let your body tell you what feels good and what you shouldn't force yourself into.

61

Finagle Your Way Out of Bed

IT'LL COME IN HANDY To get some total-body mobility work in while you're rolling out of bed.

YOU'LL NEED	TIME INVESTMENT
To be in bed and ready to start your day.	10 seconds.

HOW TO Each day, get out of bed in a weird, new way you've never tried. Dismount from the other side of the bed. Scoot off of the foot of the bed. Literally roll your way off. There's an infinite number of possibilities. Seriously, you could walk off on all fours like your dog or cat does.

62

Fill Up the Back Seat

IT'LL COME IN HANDY For forcing yourself to work on your spinal mobility while also keeping your car's passenger seat open for ride-alongs.

YOU'LL NEED A vehicle.	**TIME INVESTMENT** A few seconds when you get into and out of the car.

HOW TO Instead of stashing your bag, phone, snacks, etc., right next to you in the front passenger seat of your car, make the extra effort to load them into the back. You can open the back door to do so, or twist around in your seat to throw stuff back there. The same goes for when you actually need whatever's back there.

63

Sleep on Your Back

IT'LL COME IN HANDY To keep your spine in a relaxed, neutral position while you snooze. The result: You put less pressure on sensitive areas like your lower back and neck, and wake up with fewer movement-hindering kinks.

YOU'LL NEED To be able to comfortably sleep on your back.	**TIME INVESTMENT** 7 to 9 hours per night.

If you have sleep apnea, propping yourself up with several pillows may be necessary to keep your airway free and clear.

HOW TO Get situated for sleep with your noggin on a supportive pillow that cradles your head and keeps your esophagus higher than your stomach (because, acid reflux). If you feel some pressure on your lower back, try placing a small pillow, bolster, or blanket under your knees.

64

Stretch Your Piriformis

IT'LL COME IN HANDY To ease tight hips and help reduce pressure on your sciatic nerve (awesome if you have sciatica). The piriformis, a small muscle in your keister, is known for getting tight and, in some cases, contributing to lower back pain.

YOU'LL NEED
A soft spot on the floor (or bed) to lie down.

TIME INVESTMENT
2 to 5 minutes.

HOW TO Lie on your back, bend both knees, and cross one ankle over the opposite knee. Draw the knee of your back leg toward your chest while gently pressing the knee closest to you away from you. You should feel a deep but comfortable stretch here. Don't push past the point where your muscles start to tense up. Stay here for up to 1 minute, then switch sides. Repeat for multiple rounds if you're loving the stretch.

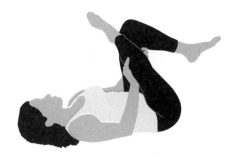

Get Down on the Floor and Play

IT'LL COME IN HANDY To entertain the kids, or fur babies, while getting a workout in.

YOU'LL NEED
The ability to get down onto and back up from the floor.

TIME INVESTMENT
A few minutes, or as long as everyone is having fun.

HOW TO Sure, you can "play" with your grandkids, dogs, or cats from the couch, but you can really play if you're down with them on the floor. Scout out a soft spot, like a rug, to cushion your hips and/or knees, and play cars, blocks, and tug-of-war.

Un-Text Your Neck

IT'LL COME IN HANDY When you're playing on your technology (always!) and don't want the neck and back deformities that come with it.

YOU'LL NEED	TIME INVESTMENT
Your phone or tablet, of course.	Whenever you're looking at your phone.

HOW TO Hold your device as close to eye-level as possible at all times. If you spend a lot of screen time at home, consider checking online for an eye-level phone stand. You'll find a ton of options, and one of them is bound to work for you.

Did You Know?

When you point your head down to look at your phone, you place roughly 60 pounds (!!!) of pressure on your neck, according to research.

Hold the Wall

IT'LL COME IN HANDY To improve your ability to extend your thoracic spine, running from the middle back to the top of the shoulders. This will help improve your posture and shoulder function.

YOU'LL NEED	TIME INVESTMENT
A wall.	60 seconds.

HOW TO Stand facing a wall and place your palms flat against it, arms outstretched. Brace your core and slowly walk your hands down the wall until your torso is as close to parallel with the floor as possible so that your body forms an L.

Stop here, and without letting your lower back arch, press your upper back down toward the floor so that your biceps run alongside your ears.

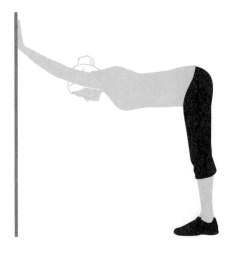

68

Tie Your Shoes

IT'LL COME IN HANDY To work your touch-your-toes hamstring flexibility while also getting you out the door.

YOU'LL NEED	TIME INVESTMENT
Shoes, and the ability to reach your feet.	60 seconds.

HOW TO Instead of sitting on a chair or couch to put on and tie your shoes, sit down on the floor like you did back in the day. Not only will you get practice getting down onto and back up from the floor, you'll have to move through a greater stretch to reach your feet.

69

Check Your Straps

IT'LL COME IN HANDY Whenever you're carrying a bag on your shoulder around town, at the airport, etc.

YOU'LL NEED	TIME INVESTMENT
A bag to carry.	However long you have that thing in tow.

HOW TO To decrease stress on your shoulder joint, whenever possible, sling bags across your shoulders as opposed to letting them hang directly below your shoulder. If your bag has more than one strap, use them, as this will distribute the downward pressure of the bag so that it doesn't cut into your shoulder. Following the same reasoning, the thicker and more padded your bag straps, the better your shoulder health.

Chill Like a Child

IT'LL COME IN HANDY At the end of a workout or throughout the day to release tension in the lower back, hips, and shoulders.

YOU'LL NEED	TIME INVESTMENT
A comfortable spot on the floor or your bed.	1 minute, although you might find yourself wanting to hang out longer.

HOW TO Bend your knees and sit on your heels with your shins resting on the bed. Fold forward over your thighs and completely relax, with your arms extended in front of you. Hold for as long as you want, and when you're ready to come out, gently sit up.

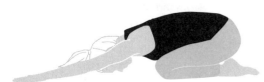

Clean Out Nooks and Crannies

IT'LL COME IN HANDY When it's time to clear grime from the baseboards, overhead fans, and blinds—and rust from your joints.

YOU'LL NEED	TIME INVESTMENT
The ability to get down on the floor, up on a step stool, and into all of those little places where dirt loves to hide.	This one might take a while, so break it up into 30-minute stints if it helps.

HOW TO Get into your spring (or any-season) cleaning, remembering that you are getting in a fantastic workout. Apart from getting your heart rate up and working your muscles, those deep cleaning motions work mobility in virtually every joint throughout your body.

72

Don't Bounce

IT'LL COME IN HANDY To get the greatest flexibility benefits from your static stretching.

YOU'LL NEED	TIME INVESTMENT
Whatever you already have to stretch.	A few minutes.

HOW TO When performing traditional bend-and-hold stretches, resist the urge to try to bounce deeper into the stretch. Doing so increases your risk of injury while actually decreasing flexibility. Every time you bounce, your nervous system recognizes a potential injury and guards the muscle by shutting it down. Instead focus on applying continuous, gentle pressure and breathing deeply to relax your nervous system into it.

73

Check Your Pee

IT'LL COME IN HANDY To make sure your muscles are well hydrated. Hydration is critical to muscle flexibility and joint mobility!

YOU'LL NEED	TIME INVESTMENT
To not get grossed out peeking into the toilet after you go.	A second.

HOW TO Keep tabs on your urine color. Barring health issues, medications, or foods like beets, if you're well hydrated, your urine will be a pale straw color. The darker yellow it is, the greater your muscles' and joints' need for fluids.

Soak in the Tub

IT'LL COME IN HANDY To relax tight muscles and aid in exercise recovery.

YOU'LL NEED	TIME INVESTMENT
A bathtub, although a stand-up shower will work in a pinch.	20 minutes.

HOW TO Following exercise or before bed, spend some time relaxing in a warm bath. While cold baths can also help with recovery, warm baths are way more comfortable and relaxing. Plus, since they temporarily increase core body temperature, they are ideal for helping reduce the amount of time it takes for you to fall asleep.

Listen to Aches and Pains

IT'LL COME IN HANDY To identify and address small flexibility and mobility issues before they become big ones.

YOU'LL NEED	TIME INVESTMENT
To become well-attuned to your body, which takes more practice than you might think.	A few seconds several times throughout the day.

HOW TO Every day and moment, your body will feel slightly different. That's okay and a natural part of life. Your job is to notice the small differences—tightness, knots, etc.—and respond by giving your body what it needs to feel better. Sit down, place your feet flat on the floor, close your eyes, and breathe slowly and deeply. Scan your body from your feet all the way up to the crown of your head, looking for areas that are holding tension or gently prodding you for attention.

Open your eyes, and give those areas your attention. Consider this chapter your toolbox.

CHAPTER 3
MUSCULAR STRENGTH

Your muscles are about way more than flexing! And they are more important to your overall health and fitness than you've likely ever thought possible. In fact, recent studies show that how much muscle you have on your frame is tightly linked to how long you'll live—and how healthy those years will be. Muscle health is even more accurate at predicting your longevity than your body mass index (your height-to-weight ratio) or your blood pressure! Yep. Your muscles are that important.

Unfortunately, muscle strength and mass begin to decline as early as age thirty, and, according to research, roughly one out of every three adults ages sixty and older has a severe form of age-related muscle loss called sarcopenia. This muscle loss can contribute to fat gain and associated illnesses, poor mobility, reduced quality of life, and even death. For example, patients undergoing surgeries or treatments for age-related conditions such as cancer have stronger, healthier outcomes and recoveries if they entered treatment with healthy levels of muscle.

Take notice, but don't let that get you down. You can effectively maintain and build muscle no matter your age! The key is to incorporate regular strength-based training into your days, focusing on exercises that will give you the biggest bang for your buck by training your body's natural movement patterns: the hip hinge, squat, lunge, push, pull, carry, and rotate.

Not sure exactly how to make that happen? You've come to the right chapter!

1

Move Free Weights

IT'LL COME IN HANDY To strengthen your body without having to hop on (and, usually, sit at) the gym's machines, while also improving your balance and total-body stability in more real-to-life movements.

YOU'LL NEED	TIME INVESTMENT
Free weights— anything that is weighted and that you can pick up and move freely.	However long or little as you want!

While dumbbells are a common example of free weights, everything from water bottles to grocery bags qualify as free weights, so get creative!

HOW TO Keep reading; this chapter contains detailed instructions on fundamental free-weight moves that you can perform wherever, whenever.

2

Squeeze Silly Putty

IT'LL COME IN HANDY To build finger and grip strength while you watch TV.

YOU'LL NEED	TIME INVESTMENT
Silly Putty and a free hand.	See if you can hold out for a few minutes per hand.

HOW TO Plop a ball of Silly Putty in one hand and start kneading. It's much harder than you might imagine!

Did You Know?

Grip strength is a great marker for overall strength—and all of the health benefits that come with it! Research even links grip strength to improved cognitive health as well as a longer lifespan.

Sit and Stand

IT'LL COME IN HANDY So that you never have to grunt your way off of the couch or toilet. It gives your hips and thighs the strength that, as you age, you'll need to help you stay functional and independent.

YOU'LL NEED	TIME INVESTMENT
A sturdy chair, bench, or couch.	A few seconds here and there.

HOW TO Take a strong tripod stance in front of a chair with your feet between hip- and shoulder-width apart and about 6 inches in front of the chair. Brace your core.

From here, slowly bend your knees and hips to lower onto the chair. Pause, then drive through your legs to return to stand. Resist the urge to use your hands or rock your torso for momentum.

Take It Further!

If this move feels too easy, rest assured that doing it on one leg at a time definitely won't! Start by lowering to the chair with one foot planted on the floor. Once your hips are resting on the chair, place both feet on the floor and rise to standing that way. Eventually, you'll be able to both lower and rise back up with only one foot on the floor!

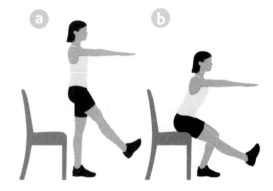

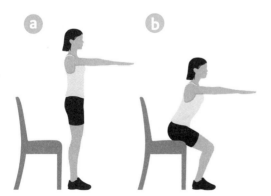

Do Kitchen-Counter Push-Ups

IT'LL COME IN HANDY To strengthen your chest, shoulders, triceps, and core when you're in the kitchen, waiting for the microwave to chime.

YOU'LL NEED
A few square feet of clean kitchen counter space; athletic shoes or grippy socks.

TIME INVESTMENT
As little or as long as you've got! You'll feel this after just a few seconds!

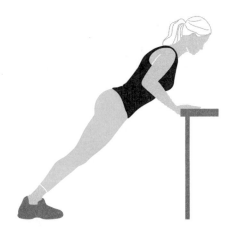

HOW TO Stand facing the kitchen counter and place your hands on its edge, just farther than shoulder-width apart. Your elbows should be straight, but not locked. Step your feet behind you so that your arms and body are completely straight, forming a 90-degree angle with each other. Brace your core and pull your shoulder blades down and back away from your ears.

From here, while inhaling, bend your elbows to lower your chest to the edge of the counter. (If, when you lower, the edge of the counter is close to your throat or face, you need to scoot forward.) Allow your elbows to flare out diagonally from your body. Pause, then exhale as you press through your hands to return to start. Repeat.

Take It Further!

If the counter becomes too easy for you, try performing with your hands on a lower surface, such as the kitchen table. If you decide to perform push-ups with your hands on the floor, please wash your hands before handling food!

5

Do the Deadlift

IT'LL COME IN HANDY To build strength through the biggest muscle groups, including your glutes, hamstrings, and lats. Plus, it can ease back pain by strengthening the muscles that support the spine while also teaching you how to "lift with your legs and not your back."

YOU'LL NEED Something to lift off of the floor, such as a dumbbell, suitcase, or laundry basket.

TIME INVESTMENT 5 minutes. However, to keep good form, take rest breaks. So you might only perform 10 or 20 reps in that time.

Yes, this is a free-weight exercise, and arguably the best one ever.

HOW TO Take a tripod stance with a weighted object resting on the floor between the balls of your feet. Brace your core. Push your hips behind you like you're trying to close a door without using your hands. Your knees will bend slightly, but only as much as is necessary for your hips to really get back. Continue pushing your hips back until you can reach the object with both hands.

Pin your shoulders down and back to tense your back, then drive through your feet to raise to standing so that the object is hanging in front of you at arms' length.

Focus on keeping your back flat throughout. Avoid any dipping in your lower back or arching in your upper back. Also, make sure your hips power the movement. You are lifting the object by pressing the floor away from you as opposed to pulling with your arms.

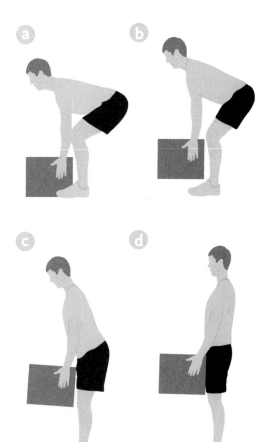

6

Raise Your Hips

IT'LL COME IN HANDY For strengthening your body's single-largest muscle group: your glutes.

YOU'LL NEED	TIME INVESTMENT
A sturdy bench or couch that's roughly knee-height.	2 to 3 minutes.

HOW TO Sit on the floor with your upper back against the edge of a bench. Position your feet flat on the floor about a foot in front of you, spread hip-width apart. Brace your core, then place your hands on the back of your head to support your neck and fix your eyes on the wall in front of you. You'll keep your face pointed toward the wall at all times.

From here, squeeze your glutes and push through your heels to raise your hips until your body forms a straight line from your knees to shoulders. Pause, then slowly lower your hips back to the floor and repeat.

The goal of this exercise is to really zone in on your glutes. If you feel it primarily in your quads, step your feet a few more inches from your body. If your hammies are burning, step your feet a few inches closer to your body.

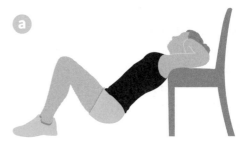

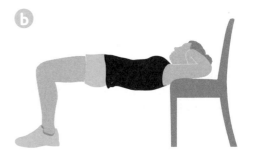

Take It Further!

Perform the hack with a mini band looped around your thighs, just above your knees. To keep the band from pulling your knees together, you will have to fire your glutes that much harder!

7

Sit Against the Wall

IT'LL COME IN HANDY To build isometric (hold it right there!) strength through your hips and thighs. This is especially great if you have cranky knees and the up-and-down motion of squats aggravates your joints.

YOU'LL NEED	**TIME INVESTMENT**
A clear, you-sized spot on a wall.	At first, as little as 5 seconds. Work up to 30-second holds as you grow stronger. Do it while you're brushing your teeth, waiting for the train, whatever!

HOW TO Lean your back against a wall and step your feet about 1 to 2 feet in front of you, spread between hip- and shoulder-width apart. Brace your core, then bend at the hips and knees to slide your back down the wall until you're sitting in an invisible chair. Only lower as far as you feel comfortable. (Eventually, you'll have to get back up!)

Hold this position as long as you can without breaking form or needing to lean your torso forward onto your thighs. That's your cue to return to standing.

8

Take the Stairs

IT'LL COME IN HANDY To build the hip and thigh strength necessary to *not* get winded by every staircase that comes your way.

YOU'LL NEED	**TIME INVESTMENT**
A staircase, but an escalator can work in a pinch.	15 to 30 seconds at a time.

HOW TO Keep a policy of skipping the elevator in favor of taking the stairs. Escalators aren't ideal, but if it's the only option and you have good coordination, go ahead and walk up the moving escalator. The left side is for walking and passing; the right is for standing. For safety, always keep your hand on or close to the railing.

9

Open Doors

IT'LL COME IN HANDY For keeping your upper-body muscles a little more active throughout the day with incredibly little effort. Any opportunity to remove automation from your routine is a win!

YOU'LL NEED
A door you need to pass through.

TIME INVESTMENT
A few seconds.

HOW TO Push, pull; you know the drill. Avoid automated doors—or make a game of trying to push automated ones faster than they are programmed to open.

10

Double Your Squats

IT'LL COME IN HANDY To get a ton of leg-strengthening squats into your day without really noticing.

YOU'LL NEED
To be able to perform the sit and stand.

TIME INVESTMENT
1 second here and there.

HOW TO Every time you lower into a squat—to sit in your desk chair, on the couch, at the dining table, or even on the toilet—rise back up and perform one more for good measure.

Tip!

During bodyweight exercises, slow down each movement or increase your range of motion. It won't make things heavier, per se, but it will increase the amount of good stress that you place on your muscles.

11

Lift Heavier

IT'LL COME IN HANDY For building more strength and health-promoting muscle with every exercise.

YOU'LL NEED	TIME INVESTMENT
Heavy objects around the house, a "heavy" resistance band, or dumbbells that weigh more than 3 pounds.	However long you were already planning to spend exercising.

If you perform a given exercise with a heavier weight, you'll feel the burn and get stronger in less time!

HOW TO When performing any strengthening exercise, do so using a resistance level that you find challenging. For example, if you're performing biceps curls with light weights, you might need to complete 20-plus reps to really work your muscles. But, if you use heavier weights, your muscles might be fully worked after 8 or 10.

When using resistance bands, make things "heavier" by using a tighter band, standing farther away from the band's anchor point, or placing your hands closer together. This will work your muscles harder.

12

Brace Through Red Lights

IT'LL COME IN HANDY For strengthening your deep-lying core muscles when you're sitting at traffic stops.

YOU'LL NEED	TIME INVESTMENT
A car and a traffic light.	Until traffic starts moving.

HOW TO Remember how you learned to brace your core back in hack 2 of Chapter 1? Do just that from a seated position. Squeeze your abs to tilt your ribs down away from the steering wheel and toward the floorboards, and flatten out the curve in the small of your back. Breathe deeply while holding this position.

13

Break Up Binge-Watching

IT'LL COME IN HANDY To add some muscle-strengthening movement to otherwise sedentary TV time.

YOU'LL NEED	TIME INVESTMENT
Nothing, except to be watching TV.	1 minute.

HOW TO Every time a streaming site asks "Are you still watching?" or a commercial break comes on, perform a bodyweight exercise of your choice. Think: countertop push-ups, squats, hip thrusts, or whatever else strikes your fancy.

14

Use a Backpack

IT'LL COME IN HANDY For strengthening your core and adding a muscle-strengthening challenge to running errands, shopping, or walking around town.

YOU'LL NEED	TIME INVESTMENT
A well-fitting backpack with support straps.	However long you're out and about.

One backpack strap should fasten around the chest and one should fasten around the waist. The straps will keep things friendly on your lower back.

HOW TO Make a habit of wearing a backpack wherever you go. Keep it stocked with a refillable water bottle, healthy snacks, and anything else you might need—and that adds some weight to the bag.

If you're going shopping, make sure to wear a big bag so that you'll have plenty of room for purchases.

15

Split Your Squats

IT'LL COME IN HANDY For putting your quads and glutes to work and upping the ante on regular squats.

YOU'LL NEED
To be able to easily perform bodyweight squats as well as single-leg stands.

TIME INVESTMENT
2 to 3 minutes.

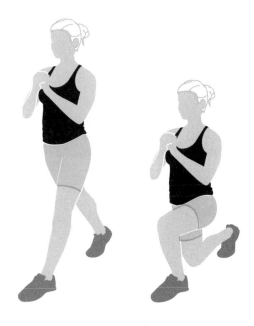

HOW TO Get in a large split stance with one leg far in front of the other, legs spread hip-width apart. Let the heel of your rear foot raise off of the floor, and shift all of your weight to your front foot. Hold your hands in front of your chest or place a hand on a sturdy object for balance.

Bend your hips and knees to lower straight down as far as is comfortable or until your front thigh is parallel to the floor. Pause, then drive through your front foot to return to the tall split stance. Focus on keeping all of your weight in your front leg. Perform all reps on one side, then switch.

Tip!

If you feel any discomfort in your front knee, try taking a bigger split stance, with your back foot even farther behind you. Keeping your back flat, bend forward at the waist so that your shoulders stay directly above your front knee throughout the entire exercise. This will take considerable stress off of the joint.

Take It Further!

Place your rear foot on a step, sturdy chair, or couch. The higher the surface, the harder the challenge.

16

Squeeze Your Knees

IT'LL COME IN HANDY As a simple way to strengthen your inner thighs, and perhaps give you flashbacks of Suzanne Somers's Thighmaster.

YOU'LL NEED A pillow, balled-up blanket, basketball, or anything soft and squishy.

TIME INVESTMENT A couple of minutes here and there while you're sitting and reading, watching TV, or playing games on your phone.

HOW TO Sitting with your feet flat on the floor, place a pillow between your knees and get squeezing. Press your knees as close as possible for 2 seconds, release, and repeat.

17

Basket It

IT'LL COME IN HANDY To help develop arm, ab, and oblique strength while you shop.

YOU'LL NEED To grab a shopping basket and, of course, be able to fit everything you're buying in that basket.

TIME INVESTMENT The duration of your shopping trip.

HOW TO When you could use a shopping cart or, with a little extra effort, a shopping basket, opt for the basket.

As your basket starts to fill up with goodies, it's important to keep your body tall and not lean.

To keep your weight centered over your hips, it'll be your instinct to lean to the side opposite of the basket. But, as you'll feel, if you pretend there's a string pulling the crown of your head straight toward the ceiling, your abs and obliques will get quite the workout!

18

Pulse

IT'LL COME IN HANDY To better challenge your muscles through their full range of motion.

YOU'LL NEED
To already be performing some strength exercises.

TIME INVESTMENT
However long you were planning to work out.

HOW TO At the top or bottom of any exercise, pulse up and down.

For example, during squats, when your hips hit their lowest point, simply bob up and down, slowly and with control. Or, when you rise back up and are almost in a standing position, bob up and down there.

You can add a pulse to each repetition or, after performing all of your repetitions, pulse as many times as you can.

Did You Know?

Your body is naturally able to exert more force in some positions than in others. (One reason why squats are so much harder at the bottom!) Pulsing like this helps you zero in on your strongest or weakest link.

19

Carry On Your Luggage

IT'LL COME IN HANDY As a way to strengthen your entire body on those long airport days.

YOU'LL NEED
A suitcase.

TIME INVESTMENT
How long will you be at the airport?

HOW TO For flights, instead of checking your bags, carry them on. Whether you're carrying them or rolling along, your muscles will benefit from the extra work as you maneuver through security, get to your gate, and board the plane.

Bonus: You won't have to pay baggage fees or worry about the airline losing your luggage.

20

Stow Overhead

IT'LL COME IN HANDY For both training and showing off your strong shoulders.

YOU'LL NEED To be on an airplane with carry-on luggage, which you should be if you're doing hack 19.

TIME INVESTMENT 10 seconds.

HOW TO Place your bags in the overhead bin—all by yourself. When someone asks, "Do you want help with that?" being able to say, "No, thanks" feels pretty awesome.

21

Seek Out Hills

IT'LL COME IN HANDY As a way to zero in on your quadricep, gluteal, and calf strength when out walking.

YOU'LL NEED To be going for a walk.

TIME INVESTMENT However long you're on a walk and you keep finding hills.

HOW TO Walking uphill (and even downhill) is much harder than cruising along on a flat sidewalk. Use that to your advantage by walking routes that you know involve inclines and declines.

Walking uphill increases how hard your leg muscles have to work with every stride, while walking downhill is particularly tough on the quads in the front of your thighs. Each time your feet land, it's up to your quads to control your steps and absorb the impact of your foot hitting the ground.

22

Hollow Your Core

IT'LL COME IN HANDY As a foundational exercise for building core strength and stability, while conveniently easing lower back pain.

YOU'LL NEED	TIME INVESTMENT
To be able to lie down on the floor and get back up.	Start with 30 seconds and increase from there if you want.

HOW TO Lie stomach-up on the floor and curl into a ball with your knees to your chest, shoulders raised off of the floor and arms hugging your knees for support.

From here, squeeze your core as tight as possible to press your lower back firmly into the floor. Once your lower back is in place, slowly let go of your knees and extend your arms out straight toward your toes.

Hold this position for 10 seconds, or until your lower back almost leaves the floor. Rest, and then repeat.

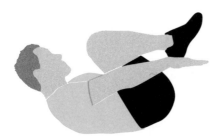

23

Test Your Suspension

IT'LL COME IN HANDY When you need to do some car maintenance and want to strengthen your entire body while you're at it.

YOU'LL NEED	TIME INVESTMENT
A vehicle.	2 minutes.

HOW TO Place your hands on the bumper and give it a push downward. Take a staggered stance so that you're leaning slightly in toward the car and your arms are extended. Bend your knees and hips to lower your entire body, pressing down straight into the bumper as you do so. You'll get your oomph not from your arms, but from your entire body working as a cohesive unit.

Go ahead and bounce all four corners of the car for good measure.

24

Rearrange Your Furniture

IT'LL COME IN HANDY For a massive total-body strength workout and a nice change of scenery.

YOU'LL NEED	TIME INVESTMENT
To be able to safely and comfortably perform deadlifts with heavy objects. You'll also need to want your furniture in new spots.	Depending on how much you want to move (and how many dust bunnies you find under the love seat) this could take from minutes to hours.

HOW TO Have you been wanting to switch up your furniture arrangement? You don't have to wait on anyone to do it for you—go ahead and make it happen.

When moving heavy or awkward objects, the key is to always lift using a deadlift. Get in close to the object, brace your core, push your hips back, and use your arms as ropes. Focus on keeping a strong torso and, as you stand up, not leaning your shoulders back.

If you need help, don't be afraid to ask for it, but you might be surprised just how light the coffee table feels when you're actually lifting with your legs.

25

Carry Stuff

IT'LL COME IN HANDY For strengthening your core, fingers, and grip.

YOU'LL NEED	TIME INVESTMENT
Stuff to carry, of course!	Generally, no more than a few minutes at a time.

HOW TO Hop on any opportunities to carry things from point A to point B. For instance, when you and your family are on a road trip, don't leave it up to the kids to unpack the car. Pitch in and show them how it's done.

Make sure to lift with a deadlift position and, as you carry, maintain a tall, upright posture. Brace your core to keep your ribs pointed down to the floor and minimize the dip in your lower back.

Did You Know?

Your ability to pick up and carry objects is a major marker for total-body strength. In fact, carry exercises are a huge part of strength competitions!

26

Make Use of Elevator Rides

IT'LL COME IN HANDY When you can't take the stairs and still want to strengthen up between floors.

YOU'LL NEED	TIME INVESTMENT
An elevator, preferably with no one else in it.	A few seconds to 1 minute.

HOW TO As you ride, perform some bodyweight lunges, squats, or biceps curls with whatever you've got in tow.

27

Pinch Books

IT'LL COME IN HANDY To work your finger and grip strength like crazy!

YOU'LL NEED	TIME INVESTMENT
Two books. Start with thin paperbacks and work your way up to thick, heavy hardbacks.	30 seconds to a few minutes.

HOW TO Position two books with their spines together, and grab them between the thumb and forefingers of one hand. Hold them at arm's length as long as you can, then try on your other side.

28

Try the Fire-Hydrant Kick

IT'LL COME IN HANDY For strengthening your glutes, improving hip stability, and shaping your backside.

YOU'LL NEED A soft space on the floor and a mini looped resistance band with a light level of resistance.

TIME INVESTMENT 5 minutes.

HOW TO Get on all fours, place a mini looped resistance band around your thighs, just above your knees, and brace your core so you're in a strong tabletop position.

From here, raise one knee straight out to the side as far as you can without dumping into your other hip, pause, then lower your knee back to the floor.

Once your knee reaches the floor, kick your heel behind you and toward the ceiling as high as possible. Pause, then lower to start and repeat. Perform all reps on one side, then the other.

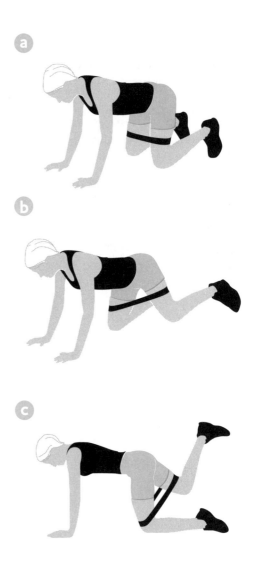

Tip!

If the exercise feels too hard, or you don't have a band with you, perform it using just your body weight.

29

Bow Good Morning

IT'LL COME IN HANDY To strengthen your spinal erector muscles, helping to protect your spine and prevent lower back maladies.

YOU'LL NEED	TIME INVESTMENT
Nothing.	30 seconds.

HOW TO Stand tall with your feet hip-width apart, place your hands on the back of your head or folded together in front of you, and brace your core. Allowing the slightest bend in your knees, push your hips back and bow your chest forward as far as is comfortable or until it's parallel to the floor. Pause, then raise back up to start and repeat. Move slowly and with purpose. You should not feel lower back pain.

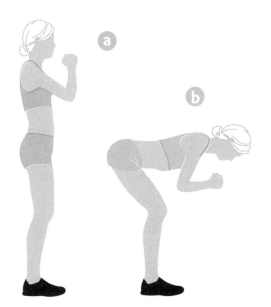

30

Wear Ankle Weights

IT'LL COME IN HANDY When you're walking around the house or out in public with wide-leg pants, wearing old-school ankle weights can add strength to your ankle, calf, and shin muscles while also increasing how hard your thighs and hips have to work with every step.

YOU'LL NEED	TIME INVESTMENT
Velcro ankle weights.	A few minutes to buy or make the weights, and then however long you're comfort-able wearing them around.

If you're crafty, use long tube socks and small, weighted objects like dried beans, quarters, etc. Place all of the weighted objects in the center of the sock and tie off both ends with rubber bands; you'll have two long, loose ends for tying your weights around your ankles.

HOW TO This one is simple: Whatever you're doing, do it in ankle weights. While walking is a natural choice, you can also use ankle weights to add resistance to leg lifts and knee extensions.

31

Book a Room a Few Floors Up

IT'LL COME IN HANDY When you're staying in a hotel and don't want to skip out on your leg-strengthening exercises, this hack can be just as beneficial as hitting the hotel gym.

YOU'LL NEED	TIME INVESTMENT
To submit a special request when making a hotel reservation.	10 seconds.

HOW TO When reserving a hotel room online, look for the box that asks for special requests. Type that you would like to stay on the second, third, fourth, or even fifth floor. You can make the same request if you're making your reservation via phone. Then, instead of taking the elevator, take the stairs to and from your room.

32

Lead with the Other Leg

IT'LL COME IN HANDY To strengthen your nondominant leg when taking the stairs.

YOU'LL NEED	TIME INVESTMENT
A staircase. They never stop coming in handy!	A few more seconds than it would normally take you to climb those stairs.

HOW TO Pay attention for very long and you'll realize that whenever you take the stairs, you always lead with the same leg. Now's the time to mix it up. If you usually lead each step with your right foot (common in right-side-dominant folks), make a point to lead with your left. It's harder than you might expect.

33

Pull Apart

IT'LL COME IN HANDY For strengthening your back and shoulder muscles, with the added benefit of helping to improve your posture.

YOU'LL NEED	TIME INVESTMENT
A long resistance band.	30 to 60 seconds.

HOW TO Hold a resistance band taut in front of your shoulders, arms fully extended. Brace your core. Without bending your elbows or leaning back, pinch your shoulders together to bring your arms out to both sides until the band is stretched to the length of your entire arm span.

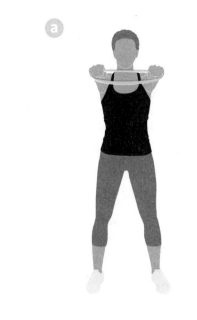

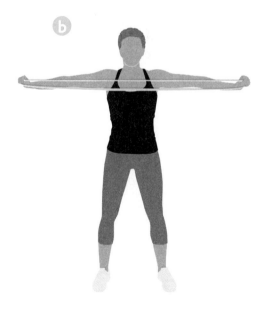

34

Laugh a Little

IT'LL COME IN HANDY To strengthen your transverse abdominis without doing any actual "core work." The transverse abdominis is your deepest abdominal muscle and helps to brace the spine; it also allows you to inhale and exhale big, deep belly breaths.

YOU'LL NEED	TIME INVESTMENT
Whatever gives you a case of the giggles—a funny video, a date with friends, a comedy show, etc.	Even a few seconds has its benefits, but once you start laughing, it might be hard to stop.

HOW TO Just laugh! It's as easy as that. Haven't you ever felt your abs burning right after—or even the day after—a laughing fit?

35

Flip Your Mattress

IT'LL COME IN HANDY For putting the deadlift back into practice, building total-body strength, and evening out that dip in your mattress.

YOU'LL NEED	TIME INVESTMENT
A mattress.	5 minutes.

HOW TO Mark regular mattress "rotate" and/or "flip" days on your calendar. Most brands recommend rotating or flipping your mattress every three months to a year.

When handling your mattress, focus on maintaining a strong core and using the deadlift, driving through your hips, to lift the mattress. You'll likely be able to rotate the mattress on your own, but count on needing a partner for flipping. Mattresses are bendy and, even if they aren't too heavy, they can be logistically awkward to flip.

36

Row

IT'LL COME IN HANDY For strengthening the muscles in your middle and upper back, as well as your arms.

YOU'LL NEED	TIME INVESTMENT
A long resistance band and a sturdy pole.	3 minutes.

HOW TO Loop the middle of a resistance band around a pole at torso height, grab both ends of the band with your palms facing each other, and step back until your arms are fully extended and the band is taut. Get in a staggered stance and brace your core. Pinch your shoulder blades together and then bend your arms to row your hands to the sides of your waist. Focus on pulling through your back, keeping your shoulders down and away from your ears, and elbows tucked into your sides.

Tip!

If you don't have a pole for looping the band, that's okay! Try looping the band around a leg of your couch or bed frame, and do the exercise from a seated position. When seated, you can also extend your legs and loop the band around your feet. If you do this, though, make sure to wrap the band around each foot a few times. The last thing you want is for it to come off and whip you in the face!

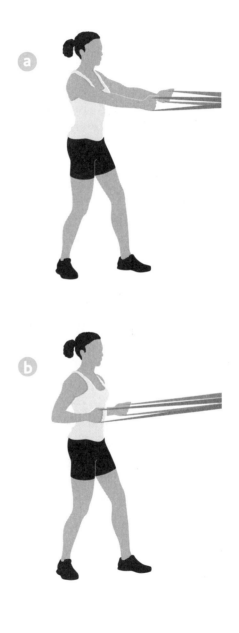

Do Anything but Sit on a Bench

IT'LL COME IN HANDY When you're at the park and want to strengthen your legs, arms, and core.

YOU'LL NEED
A park bench and stable sneakers.

TIME INVESTMENT
5 minutes.

HOW TO Use the park bench as a prop to perform your favorite exercises. Short on ideas? Here are a couple of fun ones:

▶ Rear-Foot Elevated Split Squat

Stand a few feet in front of the bench, and place the top of one foot behind you on its edge. Get your weight situated in your front foot with a tripod stance. Put your hands on your hips and brace your core. Bend your hips and knees to lower straight toward the floor, then drive through your front foot to raise back up. Perform all reps on one side, then the other.

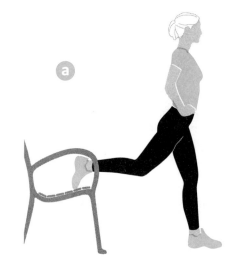

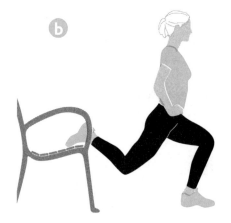

▶ **Incline Mountain Climber**

Stand facing the seat or back of the bench (the higher the surface you use, the easier this will be), and place your hands on its edge, just farther than shoulder-width apart. Step your feet behind you so that your arms and body are completely straight, forming a 90-degree angle with each other. Brace your core and pull your shoulder blades down and back away from your ears. Now, keeping everything else perfectly still, draw one knee toward your chest, pause, then return your foot back to the ground. Repeat on the other side, alternating back and forth.

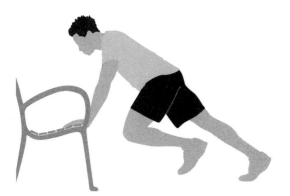

Use the Bathroom Up or Down

IT'LL COME IN HANDY To get in yet more stairs!

YOU'LL NEED	TIME INVESTMENT
Access to a bathroom on another floor in your office building or in your home.	Seconds to minutes.

HOW TO When you need to use the bathroom, don't opt for the one on your level. Instead, go up- or downstairs to whatever bathroom is on that floor.

Pull to Your Face

IT'LL COME IN HANDY To strengthen your rear delts, upper back, and rotator cuff muscles. Exercisers commonly miss these muscles, and doing so can contribute to the development of shoulder and posture issues.

YOU'LL NEED	TIME INVESTMENT
A resistance band and a pole.	5 minutes.

HOW TO Loop the middle of a resistance band around a pole at face height, grab both ends of the band with your thumbs facing the ends, and step back until your arms are fully extended and the band is taut. Get in a staggered stance and brace your core.

Pinch your shoulder blades together and then bend your arms to pull your hands to the sides of your ears, letting your elbows flare. Focus on pulling through your upper back and shoulders and keeping a stationary torso at all times.

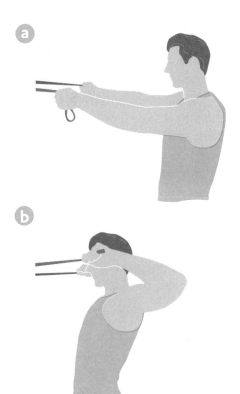

Tip!

If you don't have a pole for looping the band, try looping it around a leg of your couch or bed frame and doing the exercise from a seated position. When sitting, you can also extend your legs and loop the band around your feet. If you do this, though, make sure to wrap the band around each foot a few times. Just like with the resistance-band row, you don't want to get smacked in the face!

Do Water-Bottle Extensions

IT'LL COME IN HANDY For building strength in your triceps.

YOU'LL NEED	TIME INVESTMENT
A water bottle.	30 seconds.

HOW TO Hold a water bottle with both hands, fingers interlaced, and raise your arms straight overhead. Press your shoulders down away from your ears. Bend your elbows to lower the bottle back behind your head as far as comfortable, pause, then straighten your elbows to raise back to start. Focus on keeping your elbows next to your head and not letting them flare to the sides. Your arms will naturally want to do this to make the move easier; don't let them get away with it!

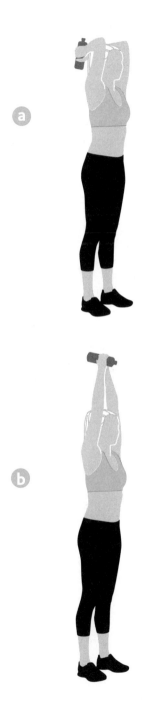

Pull Down

IT'LL COME IN HANDY For strengthening your lats. Spanning the middle portion of your back, they are the largest muscle group in your upper body and play a large role in posture and upper-body strength.

YOU'LL NEED
A long resistance band and a sturdy pole.

TIME INVESTMENT
A few minutes.

HOW TO Loop the middle of a resistance band around a pole above your head, grab both ends of the band with your palms facing each other, and step back until your arms are fully extended and the band is taut. Get in a staggered stance so that your rear leg, torso, arms, and band form one straight line. Brace your core.

Pinch your shoulder blades together and then bend your arms to row your hands in front of your shoulders. Focus on pulling through your back, keeping it neutral at all times. Pause, then slowly extend your arms to return to the starting position.

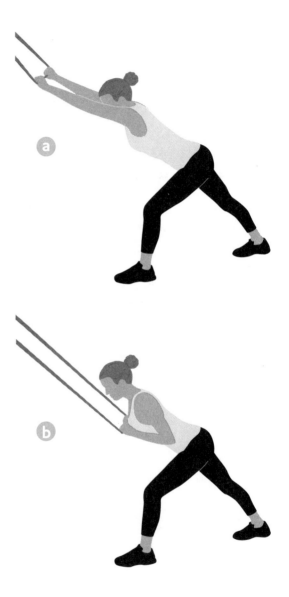

42

Shower Up

IT'LL COME IN HANDY For keeping your leg and hip muscles working during your morning routine.

YOU'LL NEED	TIME INVESTMENT
A shower, and a need to use it.	5 to 10 minutes.

HOW TO Baths are great for relaxing, but when you have the choice, opt for a stand-up shower. Every second you spend on your feet helps to keep your lower body engaged and strong.

43

Curl While You Carry

IT'LL COME IN HANDY As a multitasking way to strengthen the muscles in the front of your arms.

YOU'LL NEED	TIME INVESTMENT
To be carrying something in one or both hands.	A few seconds here and there...like when you're in the elevator or unpacking groceries.

HOW TO Keeping your elbows tucked into your sides and stable, curl your hands to your shoulders. Move slowly and with control. This isn't a race, and your muscles will work harder if you draw out each rep. Take turns performing curls with your palms facing each other and then with them straight up toward the ceiling. Each variation emphasizes different muscles.

44

Put Your Thumbs Up

IT'LL COME IN HANDY To strengthen your deltoid muscles without aggravating your shoulder joints in the way that front and side shoulder raises sometimes can.

YOU'LL NEED
Two equally weighted objects that you can hold in each hand.

TIME INVESTMENT
30 seconds to 2 minutes.

HOW TO Hold a weight in each hand down by your sides at arm's length. Keeping an upright torso and not leaning back, raise your arms diagonally in front of you until they are at shoulder height. Pause, then slowly lower both hands back down to your sides, and repeat.

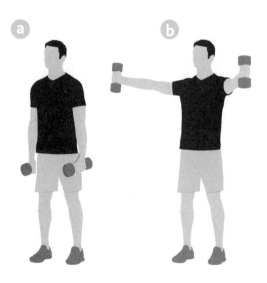

45

Hang

IT'LL COME IN HANDY As a fun way to strengthen your entire body while zeroing in on your grip and core.

YOU'LL NEED
Injury-free shoulders and something to hang from such as a pull-up bar, monkey bars, or strong branch.

TIME INVESTMENT
A few seconds at a time. When you get started, you might not be able to hang by your hands for 1 second. Keep at it, though, and you will be able to dangle like a kid again!

HOW TO Grab an overhead bar with your hands about shoulder-width apart and your palms facing away from you. Brace your core, then raise your feet from the ground and straighten your legs in front of you so that your body forms a banana shape. Hold as long as you can keep from arching your low back—and as long as your hands hold out!

46

Plank the Right Way

IT'LL COME IN HANDY As a more effective and back-friendly alternative to traditional planks.

YOU'LL NEED
To be able to perform hollow-body tucks and holds with good form.

TIME INVESTMENT
A handful of seconds at a time. Forget trying to hold planks for minutes on end!

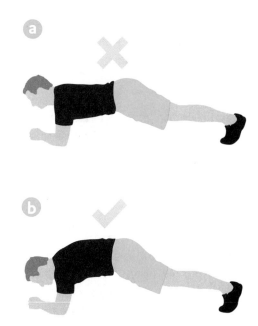

HOW TO Lie facedown on the floor and prop up your torso on your forearms so that your shoulders are directly above your elbows and your feet are close together. Clench your hands into fists, lock your knees, squeeze your glutes, and push your forearms into the floor to round your back toward the ceiling.

To increase tension further, try to touch your elbows and toes together without actually moving them. Your body should feel tight. Take slow, deep breaths in and out through your nose. Hold, squeezing every muscle, for up to 5 seconds, and then relax. If you want to do multiple reps, give yourself at least 15 to 30 seconds to rest between them.

47

Go Bowling

IT'LL COME IN HANDY For improving shoulder, grip, and finger strength without actually "exercising."

YOU'LL NEED
A bowling alley and question-able rental shoes. You can play solo or with a group.

TIME INVESTMENT
About 1 hour.

HOW TO Head to the alley and hit down some pins. If you usually roll a 6-pound ball, challenge yourself with an 8- or 10-pounder. Your forearms and fingers will have to work that much harder to maintain a tight grip, and your shoulder will get a nice workout. When choosing weights, the goal is "challenging, but doable." Always use a weight that you *know* you won't drop.

48

Play with Tempo

IT'LL COME IN HANDY To increase the muscle-strengthening benefit of every exercise—and without needing to use more weight.

YOU'LL NEED
Some patience and exercises you want to take to the next level.

TIME INVESTMENT
About how much time you were going to spend on the exercises anyway.

HOW TO Slow down the eccentric, or "easy," phase of the exercise. For example, when performing lunges, that's the time you're lowering. During resistance-band rows, it's as you straighten your arms. Try slowing things down to 2, 3, or 4 seconds. Feel the burn!

This Just In!

Research shows that this training hack can help you build strength and muscle faster, reduce the risk of injury, and even improve flexibility more than quick there-and-back reps.

49

Splash Around

IT'LL COME IN HANDY As an effective yet no-impact method for loading and strengthening your muscles.

YOU'LL NEED A pool or open water and, depending on the conditions, a life vest or float.

TIME INVESTMENT Most water-based strength classes are about 1 hour long.

HOW TO Take a water-based strengthening class. Try performing exercises such as jumping jacks, high knees, or butt kicks. The water will provide all of the resistance you need to feel your muscles burn!

50

Be a Helpful Mover

IT'LL COME IN HANDY For combining deadlifts, moving furniture, flipping mattresses, and more, all rolled into one. You'll also score major friend points.

YOU'LL NEED To either be moving homes or know some-one who is, and to be able to complete all of the above muscle hacks safely and with confidence.

TIME INVESTMENT Moving can be an all-day affair, but any time you can contribute will be a benefit.

HOW TO Speed up moving time (and cost) by unloading, unpacking, and setting up whatever you can! As always, remember to lift with your hips, not your back, and to keep that core braced.

51

Hover over the Toilet Seat

IT'LL COME IN HANDY To strengthen your isometric (hold it right there!) quad strength while conveniently keeping germs off of your bum.

YOU'LL NEED
A toilet seat. A nasty public one is great motivation.

TIME INVESTMENT
30 seconds.

HOW TO Instead of fully sitting down and relaxing on the pot, keep your hips raised just a few inches so that you don't come in contact with the seat.

52

Up Your Hairstyle

IT'LL COME IN HANDY For strengthening your shoulders while perfecting your look.

YOU'LL NEED
Hair, or at least stubble to keep neat and tidy.

TIME INVESTMENT
A few minutes to an hour, depending on how involved your hairstyle is.

HOW TO Letting your hair just do its thing is convenient, but blow-drying, styling, or even shaving or trimming your neckline is a convenient way to put your shoulders to work.

53

Press Your Chest

IT'LL COME IN HANDY As a simple, no-push-ups-required way to strengthen your chest's pectoralis muscles as well as your deltoids and triceps.

YOU'LL NEED	**TIME INVESTMENT**
Two equally weighted objects that you can hold in each hand.	2 to 3 minutes.

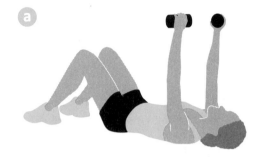

HOW TO Lie face-up on the floor with weights in both hands, arms extended straight up over your shoulders, and your wrists locked.

Keeping your forearms perpendicular to the floor, row the weights toward your torso until your upper arms touch the floor. Pause, then press your arms straight up and together.

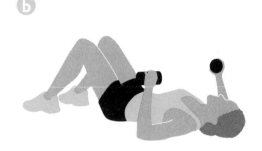

Tip!

To keep your shoulder joints happy, as you lower the weights, point your elbows down so they are at a 45-degree angle with your torso, rather than straight out to the sides.

54

Lunge with a Band

IT'LL COME IN HANDY For increasing how hard your quads and glutes have to work during lunges.

YOU'LL NEED
A long, looped resistance band and the ability to comfortably and confidently perform body-weight lunges.

TIME INVESTMENT
Just a couple of minutes at first—this one will zap your muscles fast!

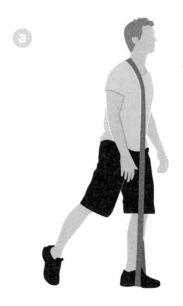

HOW TO Stand with one foot on top of a resistance band and loop the loose end of the band over your shoulders. Take an exaggerated step backward with your other foot to get into a split stance with your back heel raised and your weight equally distributed between your two feet. If needed for balance, you can place one hand on a sturdy object. The band should feel extremely tight, or "heavy," in this position.

Bend your hips and knees to lower straight down toward the floor as far as is comfortable. At the bottom of the move, there should still be some tension in the band.

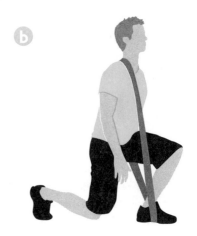

Pause, then drive through both legs to rise back up to a tall split stance. Perform all reps, then switch sides.

55

Do the Clamshell

IT'LL COME IN HANDY To strengthen the gluteus medius and minimus for better, healthier hip function.

YOU'LL NEED	TIME INVESTMENT
A clear spot on the floor, or bed, to lie down.	2 to 3 minutes.

HOW TO Lie on one side of your body with your legs and feet stacked and knees bent. Rest your head on your bottom arm. Keeping your feet together, squeeze your glutes to raise your top knee as high as you can toward the ceiling. Pause, then slowly lower your knee to return to start. Perform all reps on one side, then switch.

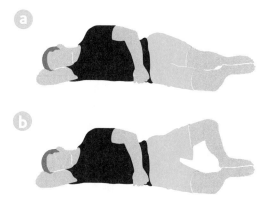

Take It Further!

Place a mini looped resistance band around both knees.

56

Take Out the Trash

IT'LL COME IN HANDY For strengthening your total body, with an emphasis on your core.

YOU'LL NEED	TIME INVESTMENT
A full trash bag that needs to go out.	30 seconds.

HOW TO No more trying to avoid trash duty! It's one easy way to add more carries to your daily to-dos. If you let the bag hang on one side of your body, you'll focus on strengthening your opposite side's obliques. Hold a bag in each arm and your transverse abdominis will do the brunt of the work.

57

Activate Your Desk

IT'LL COME IN HANDY To prevent the muscle loss that can happen when you spend all day sitting.

YOU'LL NEED	TIME INVESTMENT
A sit-stand desk, stability ball, or multiple desk surfaces with varying heights.	10 minutes every hour.

HOW TO To fight sitting disease, you don't have to spend all of your desk time standing—after all, standing in place all day isn't great for your body either! Instead, find easy ways to make your desk a little more amenable to movement and changes in position. Consider using a sit-stand desk, sitting on a stability ball that you can roll around under your hips, or moving back and forth between a sitting desk and a standing countertop space throughout the day.

58

Do the Sumo

IT'LL COME IN HANDY For performing your usual squats in a way that emphasizes the inner thigh muscles.

YOU'LL NEED	TIME INVESTMENT
To be able to perform squats.	30 seconds at a time.

HOW TO Get in a tripod stance with your feet about double shoulder-width apart and toes pointed diagonally away from your body. Hold both hands in front of your chest for balance and brace your core.

Bend your hips and knees to lower your body straight down as far as is comfortable or until your elbows touch the insides of your knees. Pause, then drive through your legs to return to standing.

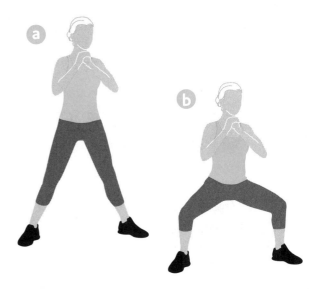

59

Pick Up

IT'LL COME IN HANDY For multitaskers! Get ready to get the house, garage, or even attic in order while giving your muscles, especially those of your upper body, a hefty workout.

YOU'LL NEED Clutter that needs you to move it to its proper place.

TIME INVESTMENT 30 minutes at a time.

HOW TO Is it time to clean out the pantry, get the broken-down Weedwacker out of the garage, or sort through all of those dusty boxes in the attic? Get sorting and lugging! Focus on lifting every object with the deadlift that, by now, you should know and love, and a braced core.

60

Press Overhead

IT'LL COME IN HANDY To strengthen your shoulders in a range of motion that can otherwise easily become weak.

YOU'LL NEED To be able to rock the wall slide from Chapter 2 and, if you want to add weights, with perfect form and without pain.

TIME INVESTMENT 30 seconds.

HOW TO Hold your hands by your shoulders, your forearms perpendicular with the ground, then press your arms straight up overhead, then lower back down and repeat. Play around with your positioning—maybe try the move with your hands diagonally or straight in front of your shoulders—to find what feels best and doesn't cause any clicking or popping.

Take It Further!

Perform the drill with weights in each hand. When adding weight, it's super important to keep your core braced and your back flat. No leaning or arching your back to make the exercise easier. If you need help staying honest, do your reps seated with your back flat against a chair.

Superset It

IT'LL COME IN HANDY To increase your workout's efficiency.

YOU'LL NEED	TIME INVESTMENT
It depends on the two exercises you pair. The example here uses a resistance band.	5 minutes or so.

HOW TO Choose two exercises that work two different muscle groups.

Perform the first exercise for a certain number of reps (or until you're about maxed out), then immediately perform the second. When you're done, rest for 30 to 60 seconds, and then repeat the cycle for 2 to 4 total rounds.

Try it out with these two moves:

▶ **Resistance-Band Row**

Loop the middle of a resistance band around a pole at torso height, grab both ends of the band with your palms facing each other, and step back until your arms are fully extended and the band is taut. Get in a staggered stance and brace your core.

Pinch your shoulder blades together and then bend your arms to row your hands to the sides of your waist. Pull through your back, keeping your shoulders down and away from your ears, and elbows tucked into your sides. Pause, then slowly return the band to start.

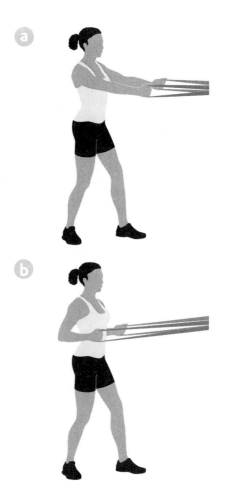

▶ **Resistance-Band Chest Fly**

Face away from the pole, taking a staggered stance and holding both ends of the band out to your sides at shoulder height, palms facing forward. Allow a small bend in your elbows and brace your core. Draw your hands in front of you, maintaining that bend in your elbows. When your hands are in front of you, pause, then slowly return the band back to start.

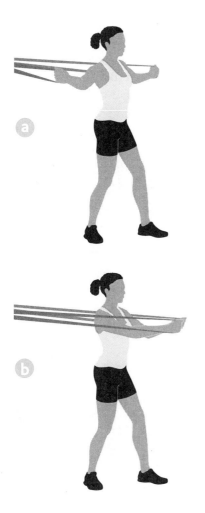

Squeeze Your Cheeks

IT'LL COME IN HANDY To keep your glutes firing and active, no matter what you're doing.

YOU'LL NEED	TIME INVESTMENT
Nothing.	A few seconds, or up to 1 minute for a real burn.

HOW TO You know the drill: Clench your butt, hold for a few seconds, relax, and repeat. Do it when you're sitting at the computer, standing at a crosswalk... whatever!

Open Jars

IT'LL COME IN HANDY To keep working that grip strength. Bonus: You'll never have to ask for help opening pickle jars again.

YOU'LL NEED Jars...and tight lids.	**TIME INVESTMENT** Hopefully just a few seconds.

HOW TO Dub yourself your home's designated jar opener. If a lid's being stubborn, using a towel or grippy glove to get more friction can help.

Curl Your Hammies

IT'LL COME IN HANDY To isolate and zero in on your hamstrings.

YOU'LL NEED A towel and the ability to easily get down onto and up from the floor.	**TIME INVESTMENT** 30 seconds per leg.

HOW TO Lie face-up with your knees bent and feet flat on the floor, about a foot from your hips; place a towel under one foot. Brace your core. Squeeze your glutes to raise your hips toward the ceiling so that your body forms a straight line from knees to shoulders. From here, slowly straighten one knee to slide the towel out away from your body, pause, and then slide it as close to your body as possible.

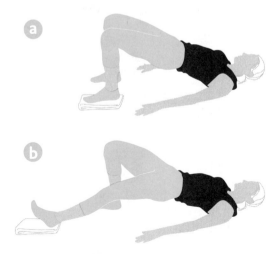

Push and Press

IT'LL COME IN HANDY To strengthen your entire body in just one move.

YOU'LL NEED	**TIME INVESTMENT**
To be able to perform a squat and a weighted overhead press. Also, weights you can hold in each hand.	30 seconds.

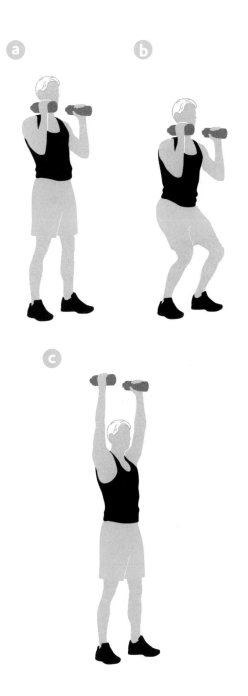

HOW TO Take a tripod stance with your feet between hip- and shoulder-width apart and hold a weight in each hand in front of your shoulders with your palms facing each other and your elbows pointed straight toward the floor. Brace your core.

Bend your knees to lower into a shallow squat, then drive through and straighten your legs, using the momentum to help you press the weights straight overhead. Keep a tall, upright torso, making sure to not arch and dump the weight into your lower back.

Pause, then lower the weights back to start, bending your knees slightly to cushion the descent.

66

Straighten Your Legs

IT'LL COME IN HANDY As an easy way to strengthen the quadriceps, in the front of your thighs, while you're watching TV, reading, or just sitting on the couch.

YOU'LL NEED
A chair or couch.

TIME INVESTMENT
2 to 3 minutes.

HOW TO Sit on a chair or couch and place your feet flat on the floor. From here, straighten one knee to extend the bottom of your foot straight in front of you, keeping your foot flexed. Pause for a few seconds, then bend your knee to slowly lower your foot back to the floor. Alternate back and forth between legs.

67

Casually Lean on Stuff

IT'LL COME IN HANDY To strengthen your deep abdominal muscles, obliques, and shoulders—whenever, wherever.

YOU'LL NEED
Something to lean against.

TIME INVESTMENT
30 seconds at a time.

HOW TO Consider empty walls, sides of couches, countertops, trees, and whatever else you happen upon an open invitation to lean. After all, when you lean to the side, holding all of your weight in your feet and one arm, you're really just doing an incline side plank.

68

Carry Your Bags in One Trip

IT'LL COME IN HANDY To see how much weight you can carry, strengthen your body from head to toe, and potentially save some time by not having to make multiple trips to and from the car.

YOU'LL NEED	TIME INVESTMENT
Lots of bags!	It depends how far you're carrying those bags, but likely 30-ish seconds.

HOW TO Remember when, as a kid, you'd help unload the car and insist on carrying a ridiculous amount all at once? Multiple bags on each arm, in both hands, and maybe one across your shoulders too?

Try it again now! It'll feel just as heavy as it did back then.

69

Paddle On

IT'LL COME IN HANDY As a fun way to explore the outdoors while strengthening your lats, upper back, shoulders, and biceps.

YOU'LL NEED	TIME INVESTMENT
A kayak, canoe, or other paddle-propelled vessel of choice—and some open water.	Plan a route that works for your schedule. Trips can easily last from 10 minutes around a pond to 1 hour or more down the river.

HOW TO Get in a kayak or canoe, and get paddling! To keep things comfy and prevent tiring out your arms in the first 5 minutes, lean your torso back slightly and focus on powering your paddle with your back. With each stroke, pull your hand down and back toward your waist as if you're performing a resistance-band row.

70

Take a Side Step Up

IT'LL COME IN HANDY To strengthen your thighs and glutes, focusing in on the gluteus medius and minimus muscles in the sides of your hips.

YOU'LL NEED	TIME INVESTMENT
A box or step—start with a short one. As you get stronger, you can increase the height.	30 seconds to 2 minutes.

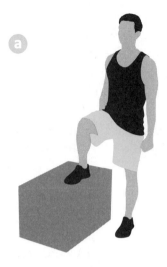

HOW TO Stand next to a sturdy box or step. Place your nearest foot on the top of the box, shift your weight into that foot, then press through its heel and midfoot (think tripod!) to raise yourself to stand. Try to minimize putting any weight into the trailing leg. The lead leg is doing all of the work here!

Pause at the top, then slowly return to start. Perform all reps, and then switch. If you feel any discomfort in your working side's knee, try using a shorter box or step.

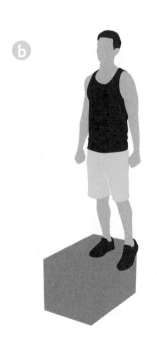

71

Give the Little Ones a Ride

IT'LL COME IN HANDY For taking your usual carry hacks to the next level. There is a big difference between carrying around an object and a live, squirming, chattering kid or fur baby.

YOU'LL NEED Kids or animals in need of carrying!

TIME INVESTMENT See how long your muscles can hold out while keeping a nice, strong back position.

HOW TO Carry around the little ones on your hips, back, or even propped up on top of your shoulders. The goal here is to keep your core braced and maintain a neutral spine at all times. No hunching forward or arching backward to rest the weight in your lower back.

72

Explode

IT'LL COME IN HANDY Plyometrics, or explosive movements, are great for building lower-body power! They're also a fun way to mix up your strength moves.

YOU'LL NEED To be performing bodyweight exercises such as squats and lunges.

TIME INVESTMENT However long you already planned to work out.

You must be able to hop, jump, or skip without any joint pain.

HOW TO Add an explosive element to your favorite exercises. One easy way? Simply add a jump! Instead of a squat, try a jump squat. Or instead of lunges, don't step one foot forward or one foot backward—scissor jump them both into place! Adding this plyometric element to your exercises will increase how hard your muscles work as well as the amount of impact on your body, so focus on getting plenty of rest, catching your breath, and letting your heart rate come down between reps and sets. Plyometrics aren't for cardio; they're for building strength and power.

73

Wipe the Windshield

IT'LL COME IN HANDY To strengthen your abs and obliques, and improve your ability to rotate your torso with ease.

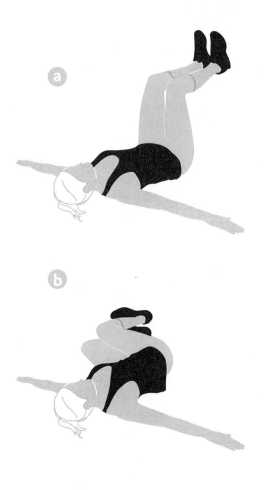

YOU'LL NEED	TIME INVESTMENT
A comfortable spot to lie on the floor.	1 to 2 minutes.

HOW TO Lie face-up on the floor with your hips and knees bent so that your shins are parallel to the floor and your feet are together. Extend your arms beside you on the floor for balance. Brace your core to press your lower back into the floor.

From here, lower your knees toward the floor on one side of you, raise them back up, and then lower them to the other side. Repeat back and forth, focusing on moving slowly, with control, and using your core to power each rep. Avoid swinging your body or using momentum. You should feel your core, and especially the sides of it, working hard!

74

Slam a Pillow

IT'LL COME IN HANDY As a way to strengthen your core without doing a single plank or crunch. You will also give your shoulders a great workout.

YOU'LL NEED A pillow (that won't fall apart if you repeatedly launch it against the floor).

TIME INVESTMENT 30 seconds.

HOW TO Grab a pillow with both hands and get in an athletic stance with your feet between hip- and shoulder-width apart and your knees slightly bent. Brace your core.

Raise the pillow straight up over your head with both hands, then squeeze your abs to quickly lower your chest, snap your arms, and launch the pillow, slamming it into the floor in front of you.

Tip!

The goal is to feel this in your abs. If you can't feel them working, focus on slamming the pillow down close to your body, right in front of, or between, your feet, and using your entire body, not just your arms, to propel the slam. Forcefully exhaling as you slam the pillow also helps!

75

Try Out Kickboxing

IT'LL COME IN HANDY As a fun way to build total-body strength—and let off some steam.

YOU'LL NEED Some stable, good-traction sneakers and either a video or live class to attend.

TIME INVESTMENT Most classes run for about 50 minutes, but there's no rule that you have to complete the entire class if you don't want to or aren't able.

HOW TO Try out a beginner or "101" class, and let loose! Don't worry about mastering every kick and jab on day one; instead, focus on having fun. While some classes involve shadowboxing—fighting with an imaginary opponent—others have actual bags that you can hit. If you have osteoporosis or osteoarthritis, especially in your wrists, ankles, elbows, or knees, the impact of punching or kicking a bag could aggravate your joints. Don't hesitate to let your instructor know if you would prefer to shadowbox with your bag. It's an amazing strength workout, just without the jolts to your joints.

CHAPTER 4

AEROBIC CAPACITY AND ENDURANCE

Most people use "aerobic" and "cardiovascular" interchangeably, but guess what? All exercise that gets your heart thumping is cardiovascular! "Aerobic" actually refers to any reaction in your body that gobbles up oxygen.

So what's your aerobic capacity? It's your body's ability to take in and use oxygen for fuel, and it's hugely important to your whole-body health. It's especially vital to your cardiovascular system's health. After all, you want your lungs to efficiently breathe in oxygen and get rid of carbon dioxide, and your heart to deliver oxygenated blood throughout your body with ease, right?

Meanwhile, aerobic endurance refers to how long your aerobic system can keep your body fueled with energy. If you want real stamina, and to tire out

less easily, you want to develop your aerobic endurance.

Conveniently, the best way to train both aerobic capacity and endurance (as well as cardiovascular health) is with aerobic exercise, or any exercise that you perform at an intensity that you could keep up for at least 3 minutes. But, get this: You don't have to exercise for hours on end to train your aerobic system or improve your cardio. In fact, in one study of exercisers, those who cycled for 10 minutes three times throughout the day improved their cardiovascular health more than those who cycled for 30 minutes in a row once per day.

So rest assured that every hack in this chapter, even if it takes only a few seconds, will improve your aerobic fitness in a big way.

1

⫸⫸⫸⫸⫸⫸⫸⫸⫸⫸⫸⫸⫸⫸⫸

Wear Sneakers

IT'LL COME IN HANDY As a comfortable way to encourage you to be more active when you're out and about.

YOU'LL NEED Sneakers, of course! Hopefully, you've already gotten fitted for some great ones.	**TIME INVESTMENT** A few seconds to lace up.

HOW TO This one is simple: When you head out the door, don't put on heels, flip-flops, or whatever uncomfortable, activity-unfriendly shoes you have in your closet. Instead, wear sneakers to set yourself up for an active, step-filled day. You'll automatically be more likely to do the rest of the hacks in this chapter!

2

⫸⫸⫸⫸⫸⫸⫸⫸⫸⫸⫸⫸⫸⫸⫸

Take the Talk Test

IT'LL COME IN HANDY To determine how hard you're working during aerobic exercise.

YOU'LL NEED Nothing.	**TIME INVESTMENT** 5 seconds.

HOW TO When you're exercising, take 5 seconds to talk to yourself or to your workout buddy. If doing so is unequivocally easy, and you can get out full, long sentences with ease, you are officially working in your low-intensity range. If you can speak in really short sentences, you are in a middle-intensity range. And if you can only get out a word or two—potentially a four-letter one—at a time, you're definitely in the high-intensity range.

Now this is important: No one range is inherently any better than the others. Your intensity, however, will determine how long you can perform any one hack. Just like a car can't maintain its top speed for hours on end, the human body can't exercise at high intensities for very long!

3

"Run" Errands

IT'LL COME IN HANDY As an active way for you to work through your to-do list.

YOU'LL NEED	**TIME INVESTMENT**
Errands that are in relatively close proximity to one another.	The duration of your errands.

HOW TO Walk, bike, jog, or full-on run from errand to errand. Bonus points if you wear your backpack from hack 14 of Chapter 3. It will increase how hard your cardiovascular system will have to work through your commute.

4

Take a Final Lap

IT'LL COME IN HANDY When you're at the supermarket and feel like adding heart-healthy steps to your shopping list.

YOU'LL NEED	**TIME INVESTMENT**
You and your groceries. Are you carrying yours in a basket?	5 minutes, tops.

HOW TO Once you've finished your shopping, do one last walk around the perimeter of the supermarket. You might be surprised just how many steps it takes!

Tip!

The perimeter of the supermarket is where you'll find fresh produce, lean meats, and dairy—many of the healthiest foods you can eat. Take the opportunity to load up on extra servings!

5

Hop Off Early

IT'LL COME IN HANDY To get in movement and steps when your errands aren't close enough together to walk them.

YOU'LL NEED	TIME INVESTMENT
To be on the bus or subway.	You'll likely add 5 to 10 minutes to your trip each time you use this hack.

HOW TO Instead of taking public transit from door to door, get off one stop early and walk the extra handful of blocks to your destination.

6

Shop in Person

IT'LL COME IN HANDY For incorporating more aerobic activity into your day while curbing your online shopping habit.

YOU'LL NEED	TIME INVESTMENT
A shopping list.	Until you reach the end of said shopping list.

HOW TO Instead of buying everything you need with a few clicks of a mouse, get up and go shopping in the three-dimensional world!

7

March in Place

IT'LL COME IN HANDY For getting in steps on particularly cold or nasty-weather days when you're cooped up inside.

YOU'LL NEED	TIME INVESTMENT
Nothing.	You can opt for a shorter workout, but how about you try for a full 10 minutes?

HOW TO Stand up and march in place! Focus on keeping a strong core and bringing your thighs up high like a soldier with each march. No phoning it in with baby steps. Pump your arms to help counterbalance your legs.

8

Bike Somewhere New

IT'LL COME IN HANDY For exploring a new-to-you city, neighborhood, park, or bike path.

YOU'LL NEED	TIME INVESTMENT
A bicycle and helmet.	30 minutes to several hours. Start with short trips before heading out on longer bike trips.

HOW TO Pick a place, find a safe way to bike there, then get pedaling! If you're looking up directions on Google Maps, tap the little cyclist symbol to find a route that's accessible via bike. You can also download MapMyRide to get cycling directions and track your ride while you're at it.

9

Add Some Jacks

IT'LL COME IN HANDY To add some heart rate–revving movement to literally anything you do.

YOU'LL NEED
Sneakers or bare feet.

TIME INVESTMENT
30 seconds at a time.

HOW TO Whatever you're doing, add some jumping jacks. Cooking on the stove? Do some jacks between turns stirring! Taking a walk around the block? Do some jacks at each corner!

10

Clean and Detail the Car

IT'LL COME IN HANDY To get and keep your heart rate elevated for improved aerobic endurance.

YOU'LL NEED
Car cleaning and detailing supplies.

TIME INVESTMENT
30 to 60 minutes. (Car fanatics will likely spend even more time.)

HOW TO Pull your car into the driveway and give it some TLC. A basic wash and detail includes washing and waxing the exterior as well as vacuuming the carpets, polishing the surfaces, and cleaning the windows.

11

Hit Up the Farmers' Market

IT'LL COME IN HANDY As an excuse to get in more walking while also stocking your kitchen with fresh, healthy produce.

YOU'LL NEED A nearby farmers' market and a reusable shopping bag. Stands typically accept credit cards, but you could bring cash just in case.

TIME INVESTMENT However long you want each week.

HOW TO Lace up your sneakers and head to your local farmers' market. Some areas have wintertime markets, but farmers' markets are the most popular in the spring, summer, and fall. Check online for the market's hours, but try to make an appearance during the first half of the day. In the second half, you could run into slim pickings.

12

Play Tag

IT'LL COME IN HANDY To get both you and the grandkids outside and running.

YOU'LL NEED At least two playmates and some yard space.

TIME INVESTMENT A good game deserves at least 10 minutes.

HOW TO Choose one player to be "it." Then don't let "it" tag you! Hide behind trees, run as fast as you can, zigzag across the yard, and just keep moving! That's the big benefit of playing tag as opposed to hide-and-seek. Tag keeps you moving, moving, moving!

The first person who gets tagged is now "it," and the game continues with minimal breaks between rounds.

13

Take the Long Route

IT'LL COME IN HANDY To get greater endurance benefits from your active commute.

YOU'LL NEED	TIME INVESTMENT
An errand to run or place to go.	Try to add an extra 5 minutes or so to your trips.

HOW TO When you're walking from place to place, but both are really close together, do an extra lap around the block or take a detour to make the trip (and your workout) just a little bit longer.

If you're using Google Maps, the app often gives you multiple route options. Pick the longer one!

14

Have a Ball

IT'LL COME IN HANDY By incorporating periods of both higher- and lower-intensity work, it'll help you develop both aerobic capacity and endurance.

YOU'LL NEED	TIME INVESTMENT
A sports ball. Soccer, base, basket, tennis—the type is up to you. If you have a fellow playmate, even better.	At least 15 minutes.

HOW TO Get a ball and start playing! You don't have to know all (or any) of the rules to get the blood pumping and have fun. In fact, the most fun game can be the one that you and your grandkids make up together.

15

Drink More Water

IT'LL COME IN HANDY To inadvertently increase your daily steps (and squats) while boosting your hydration for a healthier-working heart.

YOU'LL NEED	TIME INVESTMENT
A refillable water bottle.	Depending on how fast you drink, 5 to 10 minutes every hour or two.

HOW TO Fill your water bottle several times throughout the day, trying to increase your fluid intake to the point that, when you use the restroom, your urine is a pale yellow or straw color, a sign of good hydration. Speaking of restrooms, you'll need to get up and walk to the restroom much more often than you probably do now.

16

Walk the Dog

IT'LL COME IN HANDY To increase those steps! Research shows that dog owners walk almost twice as much as people who don't own a dog, racking up an average of 5 hours of walking per week!

YOU'LL NEED	TIME INVESTMENT
A dog! If you don't want to adopt your own (or even if you do adopt!), you can always volunteer at a local animal shelter to walk the pups.	10 to 30 minutes at a time.

HOW TO Take the dog for a walk! To make sure you're getting just as much exercise as your furry friend, use a hands-free leash. They fasten around your waist so you can pump your arms with every stride and don't have to worry about holding onto or potentially dropping your end of the leash. That said, these leashes work best with well-trained dogs that won't pull the leash (and you) around!

17

Wear a Fitness Tracker

IT'LL COME IN HANDY To help you become more aware of your daily movement habits and track your progress in increasing them.

YOU'LL NEED
A fitness tracker, such as a Fitbit, Apple Watch, or Garmin.

TIME INVESTMENT
A few seconds to put on each morning.

HOW TO Use your fitness tracker to record your active minutes, steps, workouts, and even how often you stand up and move throughout the day. Each fitness tracker has its own pros and cons, so make sure to choose one that you feel is easy to use and that you will be able to wear every day.

Did You Know?

There's nothing magical about getting 10,000 steps per day! You can still keep a goal of hitting 10,000, but if you're looking to improve your aerobic fitness, trends are far more important than raw numbers. Observe how many steps you usually take, then try to increase that number over time.

18

Cycle under Your Desk

IT'LL COME IN HANDY Depending on how hard and long you want to pedal, you'll improve your aerobic power or endurance.

YOU'LL NEED
An under-desk pedal exerciser, available from sporting goods stores and online.

TIME INVESTMENT
It's up to you!

HOW TO Position the pedal exerciser under your desk so that, when you're sitting in your chair and your feet are on the pedals, there is always at least a slight bend in your knees. Your knees should never fully straighten or lock.

Brace your core, and get pedaling, focusing on leading each stroke with your heels.

19

Take a Post-Meal Walk

IT'LL COME IN HANDY After your meals to fend off food comas, clear your head, and improve insulin health.

YOU'LL NEED
Walking shoes; a clear sidewalk, hallway, or path around your house.

TIME INVESTMENT
Up to 15 minutes or more.

HOW TO Following any meal, start walking! Maintain a moderate pace for 15 minutes; your breathing should be relaxed enough that, if you wanted to, you could easily carry on a conversation.

While walking, maintain a tall, upright posture, as if there is a string connecting the crown of your head to the ceiling. Be aware of swinging your arms forward and backward, not side to side. If your arms cross in front of your chest while walking, it's a sign that you're twisting with each step, which can throw off your balance.

This Just In!

Walking for 15 minutes after each meal can significantly improve blood sugar control in older adults with diabetes, per research from the American Diabetes Association.

20

Watch a Scary Movie

IT'LL COME IN HANDY To get in an aerobic workout without even moving. One study found that watching a scary movie can burn one hundred calories or more—about the equivalent of the energy expenditure from a 30-minute walk. The scarier the movie, the higher your heart rate and calorie burn!

YOU'LL NEED
A scary movie, and to actually like watching scary movies!

TIME INVESTMENT
Roughly 90 minutes.

HOW TO Start the movie...and start burning?

21

Sprint the Hallways

IT'LL COME IN HANDY For boosting your cardiovascular power and oomph.

YOU'LL NEED
A long, straight hallway and sneakers with good traction.

TIME INVESTMENT
The fastest 5 seconds ever.

HOW TO When you hit a hallway, pick up the pace and see how quickly you can sprint to the other end. Make sure to give yourself plenty of room to slow down. We don't want you busting any you-sized holes through the wall!

22

Go Hiking

IT'LL COME IN HANDY For views so good you'll hardly notice all of the huffing and puffing.

YOU'LL NEED
A trail. Also, a backpack equipped with water, snacks, and a first-aid kit.

TIME INVESTMENT
Choose a trail that fits your schedule and ability levels.

Hiking poles can be a great way to get your upper body working while also making every step a bit sturdier.

HOW TO Head to the great outdoors and put one foot in front of the other. Not sure where to hike? Download the AllTrails app to find trails near you, organized by length, level of difficulty, and complete with reviews and pictures from fellow hikers. Trail maps come with GPS tracking so you can keep an eye on the little blue dot.

Always start hikes earlier in the day so that, even if the treks takes longer than you planned, you won't run out of sunlight. And while you can hike solo, it's safest to always have a partner.

23

Teach the Kids Hopscotch

IT'LL COME IN HANDY To get your heart rate up while conveniently improving your coordination and teaching the next generation how to play hopscotch! Can you believe a lot of kids have never played?!

YOU'LL NEED A hopscotch board, a stone or other small object, and the grandkids or neighbor kids.

TIME INVESTMENT Roughly 15 minutes.

HOW TO Use chalk to draw a hopscotch board like this one on pavement. Or, if you're playing inside, you can place painter's tape on the floor. Then get hopping:

1. Throw a stone or other small object into square 1.
2. Hop onto the first empty square, landing on one foot for the single squares and both feet for the pairs (4-5 and 7-8).
3. Land with both feet in the 10 half circle, turn around, and head back in the same way.
4. Pick up the stone on the way back, but don't land in its square.

5. Pass the stone to the next player for their turn. Whoever completes all 10 numbers first wins!

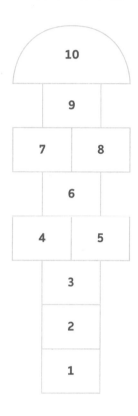

24

Listen to an Audiobook

IT'LL COME IN HANDY If you know you need to walk or jog more, but get bored easily.

YOU'LL NEED Headphones, and to download an audiobook on your phone.

TIME INVESTMENT Audiobooks often take up to 10 or more hours to finish, but you can listen in bouts as short as 10 or 15 minutes.

HOW TO Download an audiobook and make a rule to listen to it only when you walk or jog—and preferably when you're on a trail that has no vehicle traffic. While you of course want to hear every word, make sure that the volume also allows you to hear what's going on around you. Have fun, but stay alert!

25

Carry Out

IT'LL COME IN HANDY For getting in more active commuting while also saving on delivery fees.

YOU'LL NEED Your favorite neighborhood restaurant to offer not just delivery, but also carryout.

TIME INVESTMENT Up to 30 minutes.

HOW TO Don't do delivery. Instead, place your order as carryout. If possible, make the commute to and from the restaurant an active one.

26

Make a Step Challenge

IT'LL COME IN HANDY As motivation to walk more.

YOU'LL NEED
A fitness tracker. If you have the same tracker as one or more of your fitness-minded friends, you'll be able to see their steps.

TIME INVESTMENT
Think of this one as an around-the-clock hack.

HOW TO Decide with your friends if you each want to hit a certain step count per day, or if you simply want to see who can rack up the most steps over the course of a day, week, or month.

Motivate and cheer on each other! Even if it's a competition, keep it friendly!

27

Take a Fitness Vacation

IT'LL COME IN HANDY As a fun way to see a new city or even country! You'll get plenty of aerobic activity both on your trip and as you train for it.

YOU'LL NEED
A love of travel.

TIME INVESTMENT
Pick the dates that work for you.

HOW TO Making fitness part of your vacation is cool, but planning your vacation around a fitness event—like a half marathon, multiple-day hike, rock-climbing excursion, or paddleboarding trip—can be even cooler. When planning yours, one big factor to consider is elevation. If you live at or near sea level and are traveling to a place with high elevation such as the Colorado mountains, you may need several days for your body to acclimate before you are able to really exercise.

28

Get the Mail

IT'LL COME IN HANDY As a simple way to add in some steps six days per week.

YOU'LL NEED
A mailbox.

TIME INVESTMENT
1 to 2 minutes.

HOW TO This one's simple: Check the mail every day that it runs.

29

Stop Sending So Many Emails

IT'LL COME IN HANDY By forcing you to walk across the office to talk to your coworkers.

YOU'LL NEED
This one works best in your office.

TIME INVESTMENT
1 to 2 minutes per message.

HOW TO Sure, some work messages are best delivered via email, online messengers, etc., but you also need to get up and move regularly, so why not walk on over to talk to your coworkers about that big project in person?

30

Try Rowing

IT'LL COME IN HANDY To get in a total-body aerobic workout if you're not a fan of jogging or biking—or even if you are!

YOU'LL NEED	TIME INVESTMENT
Access to a rowing machine. You can find one in a gym facility.	Start with a 5- to 10-minute workout, working at a low to moderate intensity.

HOW TO Sit at a rower and secure your feet on the plates by tightening the straps across the balls of your feet. Grab both ends of the handle with an overhand, palms-down grip, and lean forward just slightly with your knees bent in front of you. Brace your core and engage your back and shoulders with your arms fully outstretched.

1. Explosively push through and straighten your legs, simultaneously hinging at your hips to lean backward just slightly.
2. Once your legs are fully extended, use your back and arms to pull the handle to your torso.
3. Return to start by slowly relaxing your arms, hinging your hips to lean slightly forward, and bending your legs.
4. Keep going! Remember, how hard you're working will determine how long you can keep going!

31

Pace As You Wait

IT'LL COME IN HANDY To get in some low-intensity aerobic exercise while you're waiting for the doctor to see you now. Because, honestly, how often are doctors on time?

YOU'LL NEED	TIME INVESTMENT
Enough space to pace around the office's waiting room without annoying other people. Or your own little exam room.	When do you think the doc will be ready for you?

HOW TO Pace! Walk around the waiting room or, if you're waiting in an exam room, do little laps there.

32

Hit Some Intervals

IT'LL COME IN HANDY For incorporating more high-intensity work into your regular cardio routines. This will help boost your aerobic power.

YOU'LL NEED To be comfortable performing aerobic exercise such as walking, jogging, cycling, or rowing and feel ready to ramp up your speed and intensity for short periods of time.

TIME INVESTMENT However long you were planning to work out already, although the high-intensity intervals can help you actually shorten your workout, if you want.

If you have a history of heart issues, first talk to your doctor to find out if high-intensity exercise is safe for you.

HOW TO Incorporate 30-second speed intervals into your aerobic workout of choice. During intervals, try to work at a speed in which your breathing would allow you to speak only a few words at a time. Once you've maintained this speed for 30 seconds, reduce your pace until you have caught your breath and can again comfortably carry on a conversation. Repeat as many times as you want!

33

Shower at Work

IT'LL COME IN HANDY To make it much easier to actively commute to work.

YOU'LL NEED A shower in your office building and toiletries stored in your desk.

TIME INVESTMENT 10 minutes to shower, plus however long the commute itself (and post-shower primping) takes you.

HOW TO Instead of showering at home, and then not actively commuting (because who wants to be sweaty and smelly at work?), sweat your way to work, get there early, and then shower!

You'll start the day feeling accomplished and energized!

Did You Know?

The average American commuter spends about three entire work weeks, or 119 hours, every year stuck in traffic, according to a recent survey.

34

Go On a Walking Tour

IT'LL COME IN HANDY As a fun way to explore a new city and get in a massive number of steps.

YOU'LL NEED
Sneakers in your suitcase.

TIME INVESTMENT
Walking tours range from 1 hour or so to a full day.

HOW TO When planning your vacation itinerary, book a walking tour. You can find an array of options online for most major cities and common tourist spots. Show up loose and ready to walk!

35

Change Channels the Old Way

IT'LL COME IN HANDY To break up sitting stints, get the blood flowing, and even reduce the risk of blood clots.

YOU'LL NEED
A TV and a spring in your butt.

TIME INVESTMENT
A few seconds...or more if you're really indecisive.

HOW TO Hide the remote! Whenever you need to change the channel or the volume on your TV, get up and do it manually. Every little bit, right?

36

Jump Rope

IT'LL COME IN HANDY For getting in aerobic exercise even when you don't have any space to actually move around.

YOU'LL NEED A jump rope, although this is actually optional.

TIME INVESTMENT Anywhere from 30 seconds to several minutes.

HOW TO In case it isn't self-explanatory, this one is all about jumping rope! Try doing two-footed bounces or, if it has been a while since you've jumped rope, opt for an alternating foot step: Step one foot, then the other, over the rope as if you're jogging or skipping.

Or, better yet—if your feet are getting tied up—just pretend that you're holding a rope. You might even get a better aerobic workout that way, since you won't have to keep untangling yourself and starting over.

37

Circuit Your Strength

IT'LL COME IN HANDY To turn your favorite strength exercises into a heart-pumping aerobic workout.

YOU'LL NEED Whatever those exercises require.

TIME INVESTMENT 10 to 15 minutes.

HOW TO Choose three or more exercises and arrange them in order so that you're never working the same muscle group back to back. Perform the first exercise for a certain number of reps, then immediately perform the second, third, fourth, and fifth. When you're done, rest for at least 30 to 60 seconds, and then go ahead and repeat the circuit for 2 to 4 total rounds.

38

Stay Off Moving Walkways

IT'LL COME IN HANDY For getting in steps and aerobic exercise when you're at the airport, hopefully carting around at least one bag.

YOU'LL NEED	TIME INVESTMENT
To be at the airport or another place with moving walkways.	Each one you skip will likely add a minute or two to your transit time.

HOW TO You know those moving walkways—the ones that are kind of like escalators, but flat—in airports? Walk right past them! Or, if you're in a rush and don't have time to tack onto your journey between gates, get on the moving walkway, and then keep walking. The left side is for walkers, the right is for standers.

39

Play Marco Polo

IT'LL COME IN HANDY As a summertime strategy to entertain the kids while getting in an aerobic workout. Between all of the swimming and holding your breath underwater, you will definitely work your endurance and cardiovascular system.

YOU'LL NEED	TIME INVESTMENT
A pool and at least one kiddo playmate.	Most games take a few minutes, and you can play however many you like.

HOW TO One player will close their eyes while everyone else moves around the pool so that they are out of reach. Keeping their eyes closed, they will then swim around the pool, trying to tag the other players. To try to find everyone sans sight, they can call out "Marco!" Everyone who is above the water when "Marco!" is called must respond "Polo!"

40

Tour a Museum

IT'LL COME IN HANDY For improving your endurance. You won't move fast, but by the last exhibit, you'll probably be pooped!

YOU'LL NEED Entry tickets to your museum of choice and comfortable sneakers.

TIME INVESTMENT Plan to spend 1 or more hours.

HOW TO Do you enjoy art? Natural history? Science? Visit a museum near you to expand your mind while putting your body to good use!

41

Run to Catch the Bus

IT'LL COME IN HANDY For getting in a high-intensity sprint, with as much motivation as you'll ever get!

YOU'LL NEED Run-worthy sneakers and a bus pass.

TIME INVESTMENT 10 to 15 seconds of sprinting to save up to 10 to 15 minutes.

HOW TO When you see that the bus is headed to beat you to its stop—and leave you in its dust and waiting for the next one—run as hard and fast as you can until you get on the bus or it pulls away without you! To pick up the pace, focus on making fast—rather than long—strides, and pump those arms.

42

Be Charitable

IT'LL COME IN HANDY To build your endurance for a cause greater than yourself.

YOU'LL NEED	TIME INVESTMENT
To sign up for a local charity walk or run.	Most charity races have a 5K component, while some have longer courses as well.

HOW TO Sign up to participate in a charity walk or run that is raising money or awareness for a cause that is important to you. See how many of your friends you can get to sign up and move with you on race day!

43

Skip the Drive-Through

IT'LL COME IN HANDY For getting in more of those coveted active moments. You'll also go through less gas, and potentially even get your coffee, prescriptions, or dry cleaning faster than you would if you waited in the drive-through line.

YOU'LL NEED	TIME INVESTMENT
To be en route to a drive-through.	Generally, 5 minutes or less.

HOW TO Instead of swinging through the drive-through, park your car and go inside.

44

Speed Up

IT'LL COME IN HANDY To increase your exercise intensity while also teaching you how to pace yourself.

YOU'LL NEED	TIME INVESTMENT
To have practice performing cardio at a nice, easy pace, and feel comfortable increasing your speed.	Up to 20 or 30 minutes.

HOW TO When jogging, cycling, or rowing, increase your speed just enough that you can feel your body working slightly harder than it was before. Try to maintain this pace; keep an eye on your fitness tracker or cardio machine's display. You can also try the talk test, aiming to stick in that middle range, to gauge your intensity.

It's likely that you'll unwittingly speed up and slow down several times over the course of your workout but, with practice, you'll get better at pacing.

45

Try Cross-Country Skiing

IT'LL COME IN HANDY To work your aerobic capacity to the nth degree. After all, cross-country skiers have some of the highest max aerobic capacities of any athletes!

YOU'LL NEED	TIME INVESTMENT
Snow and cross-country skis, shoes, and poles.	Give it 30 minutes of solid effort!

HOW TO Get set up with your skis in the groomed cross-country tracks and drop into an athletic stance, with your hips and knees bent and leaning slightly forward. Kick one leg forward, let yourself glide, and then repeat with the other, alternating back and forth. Now work in your arms, letting them move in opposition to your legs and helping propel you forward. It can be tricky to learn how to glide rather than step the skis, so be patient and, if and when you fall, go ahead and laugh at yourself.

46

Put On Skates

IT'LL COME IN HANDY As a weight-bearing but no-impact way to get in some endurance exercise. Plus, nostalgia!

YOU'LL NEED
Roller or ice skates.

TIME INVESTMENT
30 to 60 minutes.

HOW TO Strap on some skates and get moving! If you're feeling a bit rusty, go ahead and stick near the edge of the rink so you can hold on to the railing.

47

Have Sex

IT'LL COME IN HANDY For getting that heart rate up!

YOU'LL NEED
A partner and your safe-sex methods of choice.

TIME INVESTMENT
Let's just not go there.

HOW TO This isn't a sex-tips book, but to best enjoy multiple things, including the greatest aerobic benefits, take a very active role. No letting your partner do all of the work!

48

Play Paddle

IT'LL COME IN HANDY For improving aerobic capacity while also building on your coordination gains.

YOU'LL NEED Paddle boards or rackets, and a ball.

TIME INVESTMENT It's up to you!

HOW TO Hit the ball back and forth to a partner or, if you're exercising on your own, to yourself against a garage door. The one benefit to bad aim: You'll get in more running!

49

Pick Something

IT'LL COME IN HANDY In the summer and fall to enjoy the freshest produce you can get your hands on. Expect a lot of walking!

YOU'LL NEED Nothing, except permission.

TIME INVESTMENT Spending 1 hour or more on your feet, on your tip-toes, or bending down and getting back up, is 100 percent feasible.

HOW TO Pick apples, strawberries, blueberries, or whatever happens to be in season!

50

Play Active Video Games

IT'LL COME IN HANDY If you want to get moving as a family, but your grandkids are hooked on video games.

YOU'LL NEED A video game console and fitness games to play. There are a number of console game systems, and all have a variety of sports and dance games.

TIME INVESTMENT The grandkids might be stuck on it all day, so feel free to drop in and out of games as you'd like.

HOW TO Challenge your grandkids to a game of virtual tennis, soccer, bowling, or another sport. Dance-offs are also a great option!

51

Dance It Out

IT'LL COME IN HANDY To get your whole body moving and boost your mood.

YOU'LL NEED Your favorite tunes.

TIME INVESTMENT Give it whatever you've got!

HOW TO When you're at home alone, crank the music and dance like nobody's watching...because nobody is.

52

Speed Mop

IT'LL COME IN HANDY For increasing how hard your heart and lungs have to work as you mop the floors.

YOU'LL NEED	TIME INVESTMENT
A mop.	As little time as possible.

HOW TO See how fast you can mop the floor. Since you'll be moving and walking/running around at top speed, be careful not to step on any wet spots. We don't want you slipping and falling.

53

Jog in Place

IT'LL COME IN HANDY To get that heart rate up when marching in place is just too easy.

YOU'LL NEED	TIME INVESTMENT
Nothing.	Anywhere from a few-second sprint to a 30-minute endurance session works.

HOW TO It's hard to mess up this one. Just jog in place, swinging those arms, keeping a braced core, and staying on the balls of your feet.

54

Wage Tickle War

IT'LL COME IN HANDY To get wrestling, gasping for air, and keep the mood-boosting endorphins flowing.

YOU'LL NEED
Someone who really needs to be tickled.

TIME INVESTMENT
A few minutes.

HOW TO Pick a tickle fight and see who wins.

55

Take Too Many Trips

IT'LL COME IN HANDY To get in way more steps than is necessary for a given job.

YOU'LL NEED
Some time, patience, and trips to make—like when unloading the car or clothes dryer.

TIME INVESTMENT
Up to a few minutes.

HOW TO You know that whole anaerobic, strength-building, "carry your bags in one trip" hack? To work your body aerobically, do the exact opposite and carry just a few things at a time so that you have to make a ton of trips walking back and forth!

56

Play Charades

IT'LL COME IN HANDY As an unnoticeable way to get in an aerobic workout on double-date or family game night.

YOU'LL NEED	TIME INVESTMENT
Charades cards and two teams.	Most games last at least 30 minutes.

HOW TO Everyone has their own set of rules for charades, but the important thing is that you act your heart out. Move, gesticulate, don't just phone it in, and you might be out of breath by the time your group guesses it!

With those acting skills, you also might lead your group to the correct guess in record time!

57

Swim Laps

IT'LL COME IN HANDY To take your aerobic capacity and lung-pumping power to the next level.

YOU'LL NEED	TIME INVESTMENT
A pool, swimsuit, and goggles.	30 minutes or so—with plenty of rest breaks sprinkled throughout.

HOW TO Get in a lane, pick a stroke, and get swimming.

To improve your anaerobic threshold, or how hard you can work before aerobic metabolism isn't cutting it and anaerobic metabolism has to step in, focus on working at a moderate to high intensity for moderate to relatively short work bouts. For endurance, be like Dory and just keep swimming. Stick to a very low intensity to prolong how much time you can swim before needing a break.

This Just In!

Research suggests that swimmers are able to inhale and exhale more air with every breath than even runners!

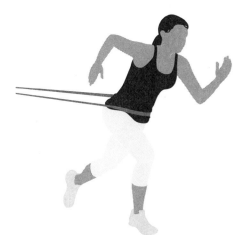

58

Run Against the Band

IT'LL COME IN HANDY To increase the intensity of your sprints and help you develop aerobic power.

YOU'LL NEED
A resistance band and either a sturdy pole or work-out buddy.

TIME INVESTMENT
Stick with short sprints of up to 20 seconds.

HOW TO Loop one end of a long resistance band around a pole or hand it to your partner. Step into the loose end, place it right along the crease in your hips, and step forward so that you don't have to hold it to keep it in place.

From here, start running hard and fast against the band. If someone is holding the other end, they will probably need to take a staggered stance to not get yanked forward.

59

Have a Pillow Fight

IT'LL COME IN HANDY For getting your whole body working and your blood pumping.

YOU'LL NEED
At least one fellow fighter and a pillow weapon for each person.

TIME INVESTMENT
Just a couple of minutes, unless you have serious play-ers who are into forts and the whole shebang.

HOW TO Grab a pillow and get swinging. Your grandkids will absolutely love this! Just make sure to first establish rules (like, maybe you don't hit faces?).

60

Play Golf

IT'LL COME IN HANDY For low-intensity aerobic conditioning.

YOU'LL NEED	TIME INVESTMENT
Your own clubs or to rent some.	It takes an average of 4 hours to golf eighteen holes, but you can go for nine holes or even fewer.

HOW TO Walking the course will let you get in a lot of steps, but depending on how many holes you're hitting, carrying your clubs through the whole course could be a little much. So if you're golfing with friends, take turns with who drives the cart and clubs and who hoofs it.

61

Take Laps Around the Terminal

IT'LL COME IN HANDY As a way to stay moving during long layovers.

YOU'LL NEED	TIME INVESTMENT
To be at the airport.	This could take up to 30 minutes or more if you do a full loop. You might be surprised just how big some airport terminals are.

HOW TO Walk from your gate to the opposite end of the terminal and back again. Remember, no moving walkways!

62

Walk and Talk

IT'LL COME IN HANDY If you want to get up and move more throughout the day, but you're tied to your phone.

YOU'LL NEED
Bluetooth headphones or a hands-free phone set.

TIME INVESTMENT
However long you're on the phone.

HOW TO If you're on the phone, get up and walk! Keep a nice, easy pace so that no one hears you panting.

63

Run Through the Sprinkler

IT'LL COME IN HANDY In summer to get in little running bursts while playing in the yard with the family.

YOU'LL NEED
A sprinkler and, if you don't want your clothes to get soggy, a swimsuit.

TIME INVESTMENT
Each run-through will take about 3 seconds.

HOW TO Go ahead, live a little and cool off with a run through the sprinkler. If your childhood memories are fuzzy, the key is to make a small hop over the actual sprinkler so that you don't stub your toe or wipe out on the slick grass. And always get a good running start!

64

Park Away from the Entrance

IT'LL COME IN HANDY For working more steps and active minutes into your day. You might also cut down on time circling parking lots looking for the "perfect" spot.

YOU'LL NEED	TIME INVESTMENT
Your car, and a need to park it.	You might end up walking an extra minute or two.

HOW TO When parking at stores, restaurants, and whatnot, choose a space that's as far away from the entrance as possible. If you're really into it, you can even park at the end of your driveway when you get home.

65

Have Active Hangouts

IT'LL COME IN HANDY So that you don't have to choose between exercise time and social time.

YOU'LL NEED	TIME INVESTMENT
Friends who are amenable to movement.	It's up to you and your friends.

HOW TO Instead of always going to dinner and a movie when you're with your friends, choose more aerobically active hangout options such as going for a walk, visiting a park, or hitting up a street fair.

66

Play with Fartleks

IT'LL COME IN HANDY To integrate high-intensity intervals with your regular run schedule.

YOU'LL NEED To be able to perform high-intensity intervals when running.

TIME INVESTMENT You'll spend the same amount of time running as you were going to anyway, but each fartlek should take under 1 minute.

HOW TO Rest assured that these have nothing to do with farts. (*Fartlek* means "speed play" in Swedish.) Fartleks are a run-training technique in which, while running, you spot an object in front of you and then sprint toward it. Once you reach it, you slowly back down to your base pace. That's one fartlek! Do as many as you want.

67

Hit Up the Batting Cages

IT'LL COME IN HANDY As a fun way to get your heart pumping and get in a cardiovascular workout without ever moving your feet.

YOU'LL NEED A batting cage, helmet, and stack of quarters.

TIME INVESTMENT Each go-round will take just a few minutes. Play to your heart's content.

HOW TO Set up with your feet greater than shoulder-width apart about one foot to the side of the plate, allow a slight bend in your knees and hips, and keep your eye on the ball! Remember, the first round doesn't count; it's just practice.

68

Mow the Lawn

IT'LL COME IN HANDY To perform intense aerobic activity while also building total-body strength and muscular endurance.

YOU'LL NEED	TIME INVESTMENT
A push mower.	It depends on how much grass you have.

HOW TO With push mowing, the key is to maintain total-body tension at all times. Brace your core and keep your shoulders firm. This will make you so much more efficient while also keeping things comfortable on your joints and back.

69

Play Arcade Games

IT'LL COME IN HANDY As an active hangout or date-night idea that gets you on your feet and gets your heart pumping.

YOU'LL NEED	TIME INVESTMENT
Tokens.	However long you're having fun!

HOW TO Games like Skee-Ball, hoops, and air hockey might not be "sports," but they will certainly get you moving, and some might even get you sweating.

70

Take an Indoor Cycling Class

IT'LL COME IN HANDY If you're up for taking your regular bike rides inside. There, you can give your aerobic workout all you've got—since you won't have to be on the lookout for potholes, etc.

YOU'LL NEED To be able to perform high-intensity exercise.

TIME INVESTMENT Most classes are 1 hour long.

HOW TO Sign up and, when you sign in, get a pair of cycling shoes. Clipping into the pedals is notoriously tricky, so after you get your bike situated, ask someone to show you how to clip in. Oftentimes, a trainer is walking around the studio before class just to help.

Tip!

You can and should ask for help setting up your bike, but this will get you started: Adjust the saddle height so it is right above your hip bones. Set the handlebars so they're the same height or just a bit higher than your seat and, if you place your elbow at the front edge of the seat, they're a couple inches in front of the tips of your fingers.

71

Push a Wheelchair

IT'LL COME IN HANDY To do good for others while simultaneously benefiting your endurance, especially on longer excursions.

YOU'LL NEED A wheelchair-using friend or family member who might like to rest their arms every once in a while.

TIME INVESTMENT It's up to you two to choose.

HOW TO Help out by pushing your friend or family member's wheelchair for the afternoon, with their permission. Or, if you'd really like to help out someone who is differently abled, consider volunteering at a hospital or senior living facility.

72

Visit the Zoo

IT'LL COME IN HANDY For getting in steps and improving endurance. And anything with animals comes with bonus points.

YOU'LL NEED Admission tickets and comfortable sneakers.

TIME INVESTMENT 1 to 2 hours.

HOW TO Head to the zoo with friends or family and have a great afternoon. Easy as that!

73

Rake Leaves

IT'LL COME IN HANDY For increasing aerobic capacity, burning calories, and building core and arm strength while you're at it.

YOU'LL NEED Fallen leaves and a good rake.

TIME INVESTMENT It depends on the trees.

HOW TO Rake the leaves into multiple small piles, then wait for help to bag them. If you try to bag them without someone holding the bag open, you might end up with leaves everywhere and need to rake again.

74

Corral Your Cart

IT'LL COME IN HANDY For getting in more steps on shopping trips while also being a good human.

YOU'LL NEED
An unloaded shopping cart in a parking lot.

TIME INVESTMENT
30 seconds.

HOW TO Return your shopping cart—or, if you're feeling generous, any other rogue rollers—to their corral.

75

Catch Lightning Bugs

IT'LL COME IN HANDY To incorporate more active minutes into your summer and fun with your grandkids into your memory bank.

YOU'LL NEED
A glass jar with holes poked in the lid.

TIME INVESTMENT
30 minutes.

HOW TO Take the kids and go lightning-bug hunting! You'll feel pretty silly darting all over the yard for little specks of light that, by the time you reach them, are long gone. But you'll have fun and maybe, just maybe, catch one or two nightlights.

CONCLUSION

Old habits die hard.
New habits take practice.

While we often say, "It takes twenty-one days to form a habit," current research shows that it can actually take much longer for a behavior to become fully ingrained and for us to execute on autopilot. After all, everything—from our childhood upbringings and relationships with our bodies to the ways we deal with stress and prioritize our time—impacts our fitness journeys and where we will find ourselves along them at any given moment.

When we understand that building and breaking habits can be difficult—and understand our triggers, motivators, and thought processes—we are better able to treat ourselves with the compassion we need to stay the course. If we start to "slip," we don't throw in the towel or label anything a failure. Instead, we simply observe what did and didn't work, and use that information to help ourselves make even better decisions in the future for a healthier, happier life.

Because that's what we deserve, and it's never too late to get fit. Promise.

INDEX

ABOUT THE AUTHOR

K. Aleisha Fetters, CSCS, is a journalist and certified strength and conditioning specialist whose work has been featured in publications including *Time*; *Women's Health*; *Runner's World*; *O, The Oprah Magazine*; *US News & World Report*; *Men's Health*; *Self*; *Diabetic Living*; and SilverSneakers.com. She is coauthor of *The Woman's Guide to Strength Training* and is regularly interviewed as an expert for publications including *Shape*, FoodNetwork.com, *Beachbody*, *Lifehacker*, and *DietSpotlight*.